Dieting Causes Brain Damage

Other Books by Bradley Trevor Greive

The Blue Day Book
The Blue Day Journal and Directory
Dear Mom
Looking for Mr. Right
The Meaning of Life
The Incredible Truth About Mothers
Tomorrow
Priceless: The Vanishing Beauty of a Fragile Planet
The Book for People Who Do Too Much
Friends to the End
Dear Dad
The Simple Truth About Love
A Teaspoon of Courage

For Children

The Blue Day Book for Kids
Friends to the End for Kids

Dieting Causes
Brain Damage

How to Lose Weight
without Losing Your Mind

BRADLEY TREVOR GREIVE

**Andrews McMeel
Publishing, LLC**

Kansas City

06 07 08 09 10 TWP 10 9 8 7 6 5 4 3 2 1

ISBN-13: 978-0-7407-6158-4
ISBN-10: 0-7407-6158-7

Library of Congress Control Number: 2006923250

Photo Credits
Acclaim Images (USA) • www.acclaimimages.com
Adam Jesser Photography (Australia) • www.adamjesser.com
Africa Imagery (South Africa) • www.africaimagery.com
Auscape International (Australia) • www.auscape.com.au
Australian Picture Library (Australia) • www.australianpicturelibrary.com.au
Austral International (Australia) • www.australphoto.com.au
Esther Beaton Wild Pictures (Australia) • www.estherbeaton.com
Exikon (Australia) • www.exikon.com
Getty Images (Australia) • www.gettyimages.com
Jupiter Images (Australia) • www.jupiterimages.com.au
Natural Exposures (USA) • www.naturalexposures.com
Nature Picture Library (UK) • www.naturepl.com
Photolibrary.com (Australia) • www.photolibrary.com
Sharon Beals (USA) • www.sharonbeals.com
Steve Bloom Images (UK) • www.stevebloom.com
Still Pictures (UK) • www.stillpictures.com

Detailed page credits for the remarkable photographers whose work appears in *Dieting Causes Brain Damage* and other books by Bradley Trevor Greive are freely available at www.btgstudios.com.

Book design by Holly Camerlinck

Attention: Schools and Businesses
Andrews McMeel books are available at quantity discounts with bulk purchase for educational, business, or sales promotional use. For information, please write to: Special Sales Department, Andrews McMeel Publishing, LLC, 4520 Main Street, Kansas City, Missouri 64111.

"I'm on this amazing new diet. You can eat whatever you want, whenever you want, and as much as you want. You don't lose any weight, but it's very easy to stick to."

• GEORGE TRICKER •

"I paid four hundred bucks to join a health club last year. Haven't lost a pound. Apparently you have to show up."

• RICH CEISLER •

"The amount of sleep required by the average person is about five minutes more."

• MAX KAUFFMANN •

ACKNOWLEDGMENTS

I have always been a man of impressive dimensions and, generally speaking, this pleases me. However, when I started writing this book I had set a new personal record for my individual mass, tipping the scales a few ounces on the dark side of 280 pounds. At six feet three inches tall, this was not the end of the world. I was well short of being taken to the hospital on a forklift or being asked to audition for tasteless reality TV shows.

Though increasingly couch potato–esque in my behavior, I was still lifting weights regularly and felt reasonably healthy. In fact, I even won a regional rock-lifting competition in French Polynesia wearing a colorful sarong and floral crown, and I looked mighty fine doing it. So at first, I was quite flattered when friends said I looked like an NFL linebacker. Then one day I couldn't zip up my jeans, and it occurred to me that I was not an NFL linebacker at all. I was just an author of amusing little books, a vocation that is not generally aided by a barrel chest or the bulky neck of an ox with thyroid problems.

Like everyone, I had my reasons for the blowout, but all the excuses in the world wouldn't get my pants buttoned up. I realized that to feel good about myself I had to lose some weight and get back into shape.

After turning off some vacuous and voyeuristic health and fitness TV shows in disgust, I grabbed a few diet books and was both horrified and amused by what I found. Much of what I read was either stupid, extreme, outdated, potentially dangerous, or based on the assumption that I wanted to wax my chest and grate Parmesan cheese on my abs. I decided to get back to basics, and this modest book is the summary of what I learned about how to look and feel my best in the most effective, no-nonsense way.

There is no miracle cure for chronic obesity or even drastic love-handle reduction, but in the medium and long term, this book is guaranteed to help you if you are trying to get into better shape—even if it only makes you laugh as you move closer to your personal weight-loss goals.

Ironically, this book is the fattest of the Blue Day Book series so far. Nevertheless, *Dieting Causes Brain Damage* would not be as buff as it is if it were not for Chris Schillig, my beloved editorial goddess from Andrews McMeel Publishing in Kansas City, Missouri, who flew halfway around the planet to help me whip this chubby volume into shape. And without my tremendous team at BTG Studios in Australia, I would soon be a wandering zombie, incapable of putting pen to paper. Mr. Mark Bowmer, my research assistant/consulting scribe/golf buddy, is long overdue for special mention, along with a stellar cast of tireless talents, all of whom are superbly wrangled by the redoubtable Ms. Nerida Robinson on a daily basis.

It would be perverse not to thank the many extraordinary photographers and their learned representatives throughout the world who have generously shared their visual genius with me once again. I encourage everyone interested in premium photography to seek out their updated contact details posted at www.btgstudios.com.

When it comes to maintaining both a dashing figure and potent gravitas, I have always been inspired by my svelte literary über-agent, Sir Albert J. Zuckerman of Writers House, New York. During the Korean War Al, then a decorated lieutenant with the U.S. Navy's legendary "Naked Warriors" of the Underwater Demolition Teams, the forerunners of the Navy SEALs, was summoned before the Special Operations Group High Command and ordered to employ his extensive linguistic abilities and honed fighting and evasion skills in carrying vital secret messages to friendly guerilla units deep behind enemy lines, in effect becoming a human carrier pigeon.

In 1951, the best way to securely convey classified material was to ingest a small anticorrosive, pill-shaped metal canister containing a microfilm message and then regurgitate it once the objective had been reached. Known as "Victory Mules" by their allies and as "Shadowy Dogs Whose Bellies Are Filled with Poisonous Lies" by the North Koreans, Al and his men braved countless dangers in their quest to cough up the decisive intelligence that turned the tide in the allies' favor when it mattered most.

Though Al's superior language skills and gift for indigenous disguises prevented him from being detected or intercepted by the enemy, each mission took a terrible toll. By the end of hostilities, "Big" Al was reduced to skin and bones. The act of repeatedly vomiting on demand had left him with a curious case of faux bulimia and his health was in serious jeopardy.

After returning home to Brooklyn, he continued to struggle, unable to stomach nutritious meals or enjoy even the slightest prandial excess without violently antisocial consequences. Luckily, just when he felt he could go no further, he found the love of his life, Ms. Claire Thompson. Claire is an amazing culinary artiste, and when she saw how Al fought to keep his dinner down on their first date, she offered to cook a meal for him. On their fateful second date, Claire produced a sensuous array of velvety, flavorsome dishes that soothed Al's visceral torment while sending his taste buds scampering with ecstatic rapture.

Of course, the downside to this delicious union was that, with the sudden surge in his appetite, Al's waistline expanded at an alarming rate and, for the first time in many years, he was forced to watch his weight. Al took this challenge in his stride, achieving and maintaining the lithe and chiseled physique that continues to thrill first ladies and terrorize the senior tennis circuit throughout the world.

Recently, when I was struggling desperately with my own considerable girth, I sought the great man's wisdom after dining with Al and Claire in their Chelsea brownstone. When we had retired to the Tiffany Room for coffee and port, I asked Sir Albert how he managed to stay so trim, taut, and terrific while subsisting on a diet that would make Alain Ducasse's arteries harden. "My dear boy," he responded gently, proffering a sumptuous cheese plate, "it's simply a question of balance. For every nibble of pâté, I take a very big bite out of life."

Bravo, Sir Albert. At last a recipe for success that tastes divine.

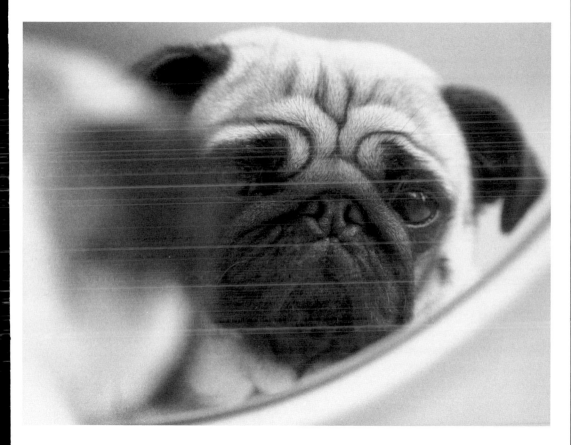

It's not uncommon to feel slightly nonplussed
when you look in the mirror.

1

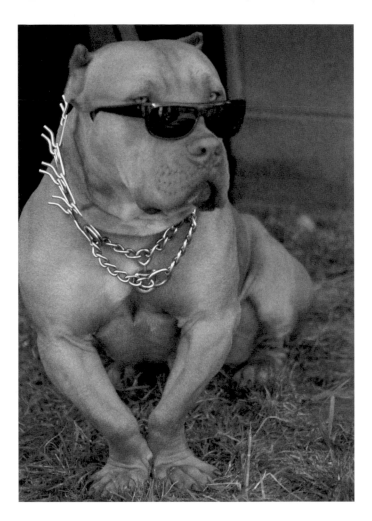

If you watch TV, go to movies, or read magazines, you may believe
that all men are supposed to be bronzed, muscle-bound freaks,

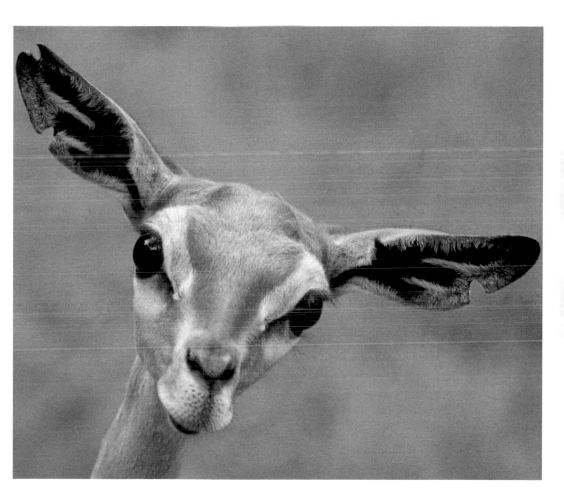

and all women should look like alien-headed supermodels. 3

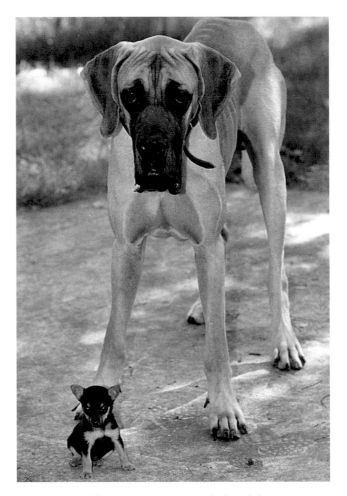

But normal beings cannot and should not try to
measure themselves against the media's airbrushed,
airheaded ideals that are totally out of touch with reality.

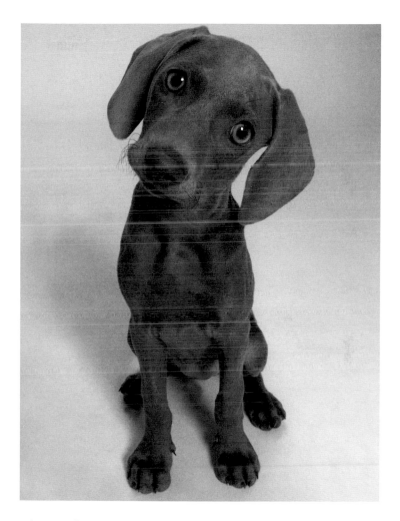

Ultimately, as we've all been told so many times, it's not how the world sees you that matters, it's how you see yourself.

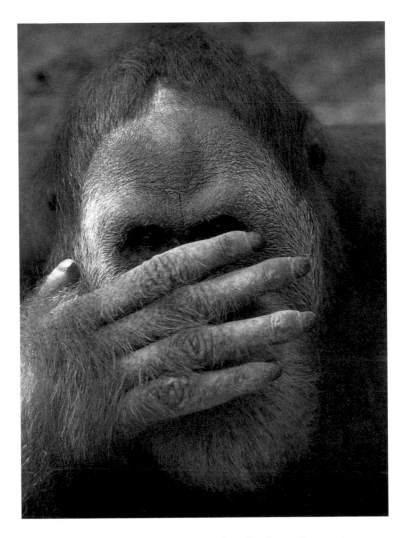

If you are often frightened to look at the scale,

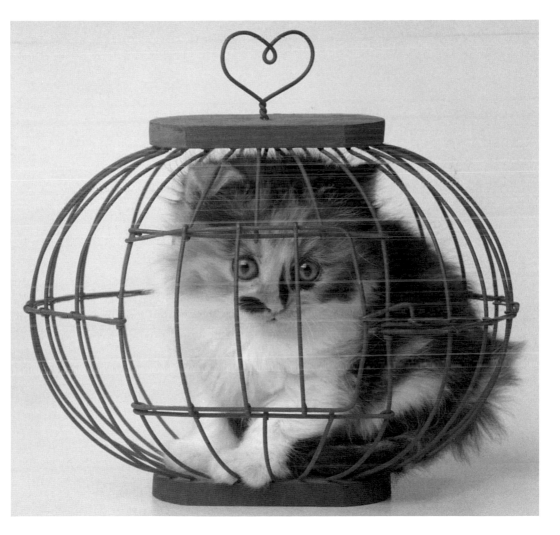

feeling romantically limited,

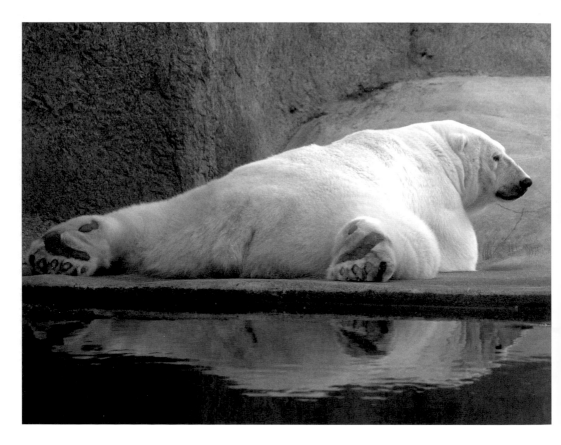

becoming self-conscious about sunbathing on the beach,

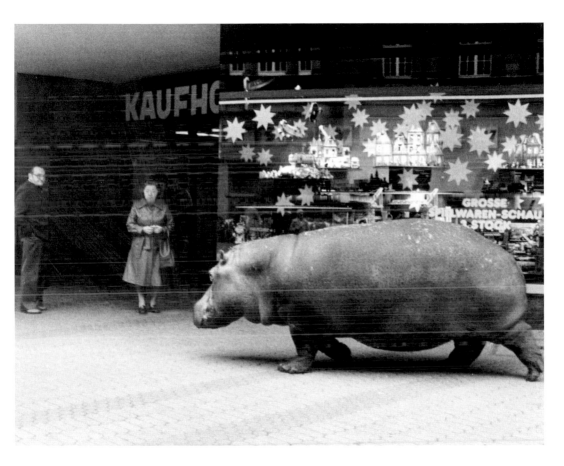

spending all day shopping without finding
a single outfit you like that fits,

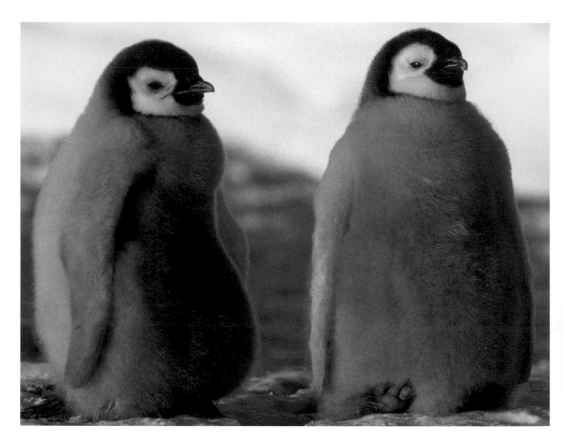

and sucking in your stomach in public—then, well,
maybe you have a genuine problem.

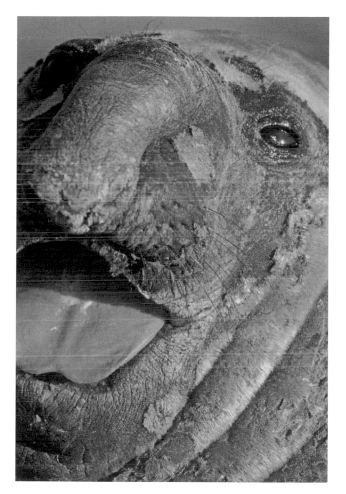

The bottom line is if you have ever felt ugly because of your weight,
you need to start making some real changes in your life.
And the time for taking action starts *right now*!

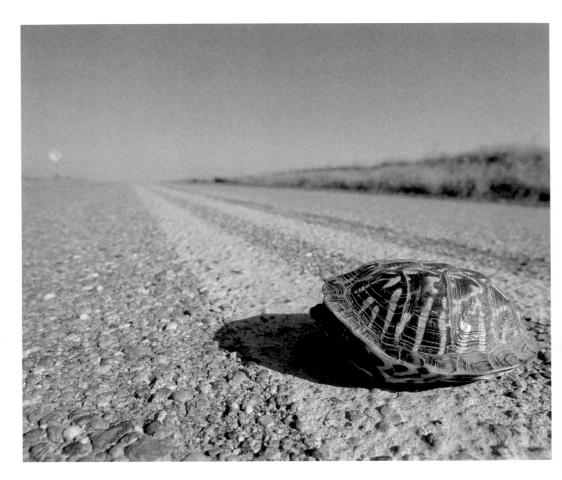

Alas, if you're like most people, you'll do nothing about it.
You might pretend it isn't happening and damn the consequences,

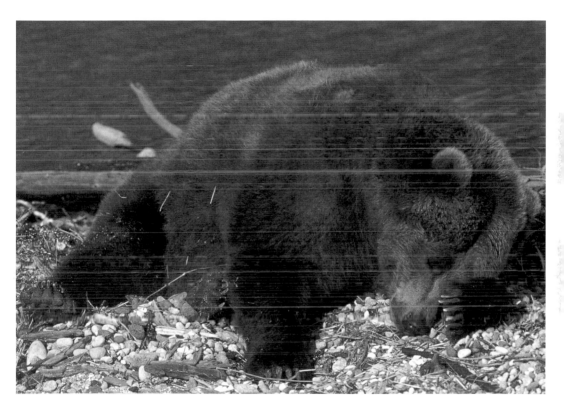

or simply become a miserable recluse
and spend your holiday weekends wallowing in self-pity.

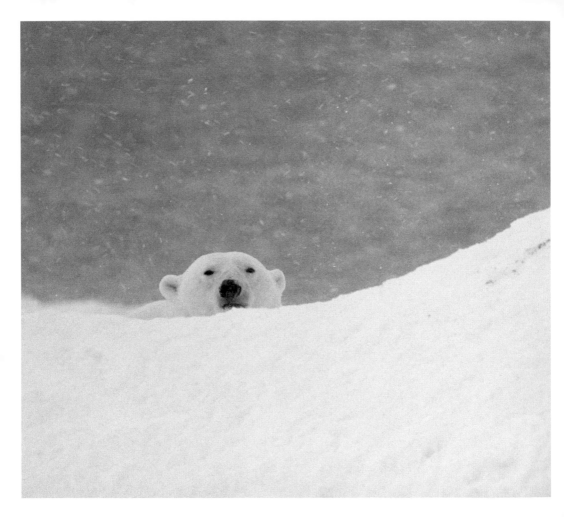

You could move to a part of the world where
a generous layer of body fat is essential for survival

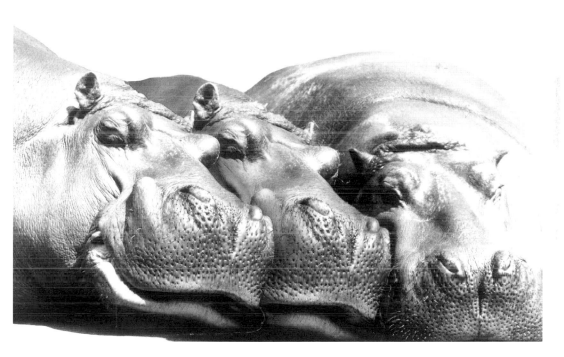

or try to make yourself feel better by associating exclusively
with people who are much fatter than you are. Luckily, in North America
these days, this is surprisingly easy to do.

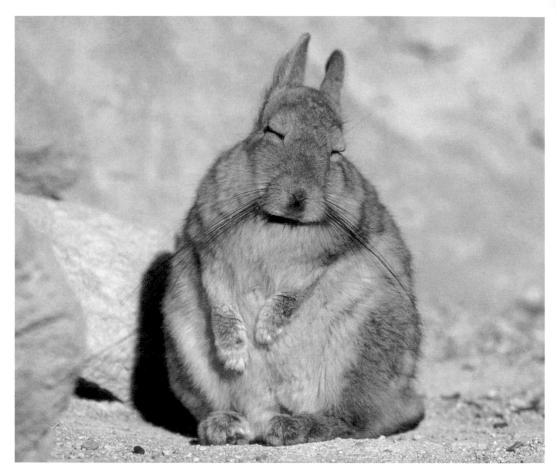

The biggest reason people don't lose weight is that they never actually take any meaningful action. They *say* they want to, but then the excuses come. It seems there may well be a direct link between love handles and personal integrity.

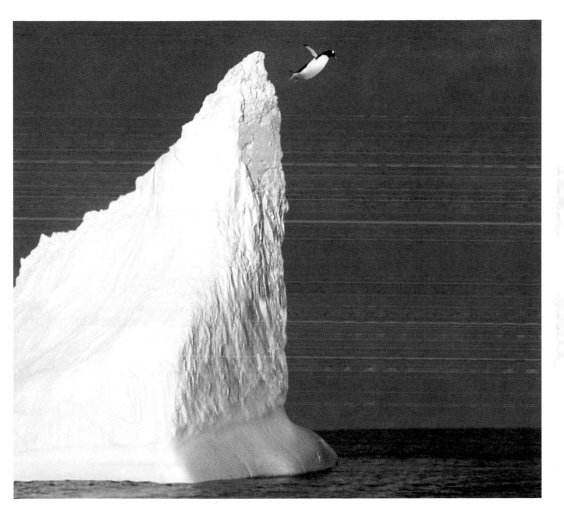

The next biggest reason is that they start out
by taking everything to extremes.

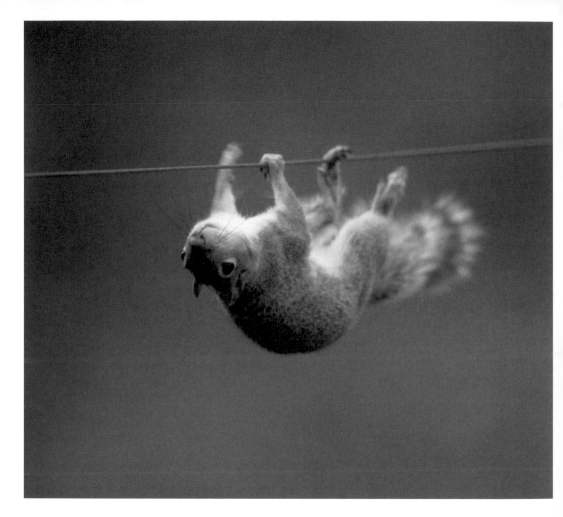

They go from being fairly spongy and sedentary to exercising as if they were training for the Special Forces:

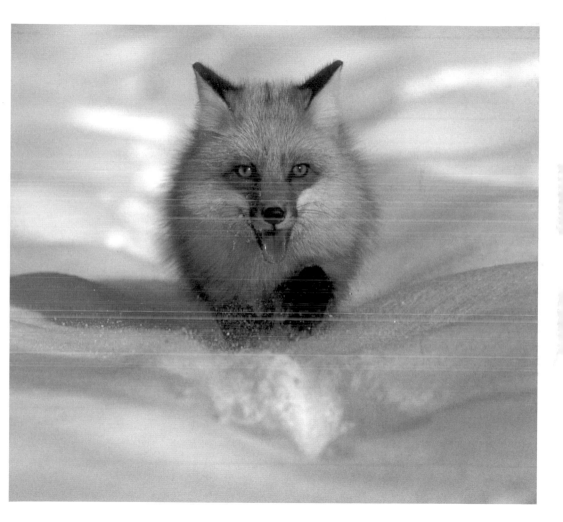

grueling workouts in the gym, swimming two miles before breakfast, and running marathons on hard pavement, hot sand, and soft snow.

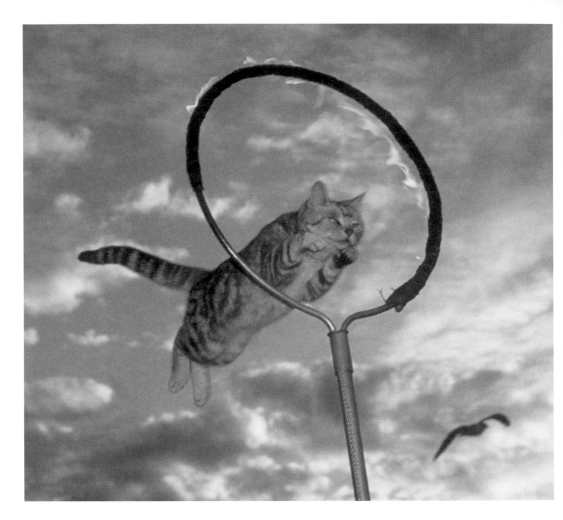

Nothing is too tough—they are going to lose weight
and get six-pack abs or die trying.

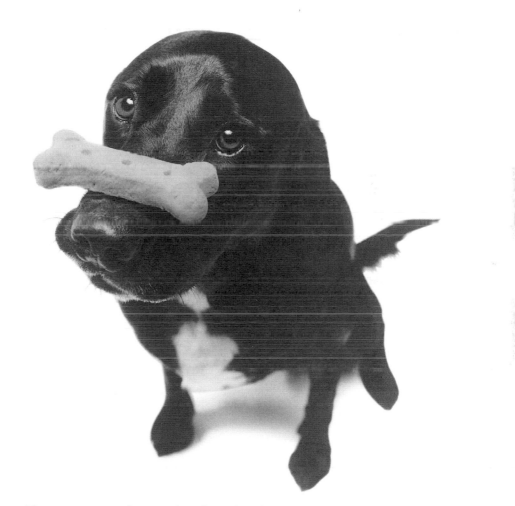

The same goes for meals. They decide they'd almost rather not
eat at all anymore. Starving themselves and feeling hungry all the time
become sick affirmations that they are losing weight fast.

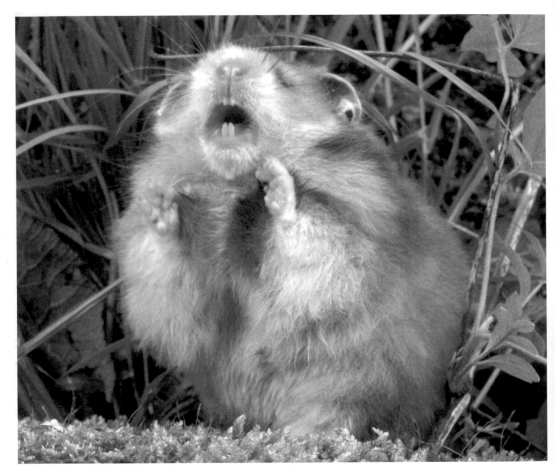

Hunger and fatigue are a deadly combination, so this regimen can only go on for so long before the cracks begin to appear. "Oh merciful gods, I simply cannot do another set of crunches or face another plate of steamed lettuce. Please, I beg you, *Smite me now*!"

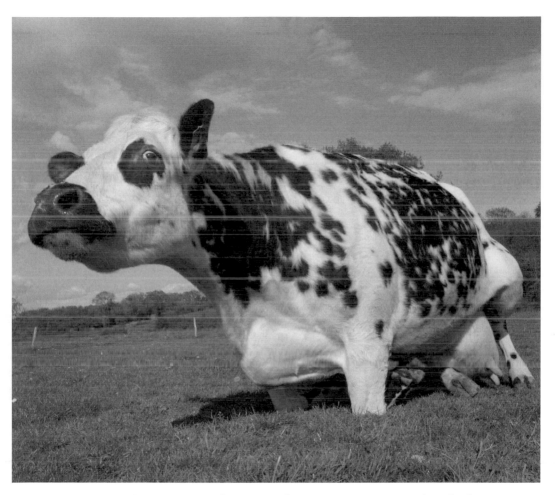

Pretty soon they run out of energy, their immune systems break down, injuries pile up, their legs turn to jelly, and finally—*Craaaaaash*! They are down for the count.

23

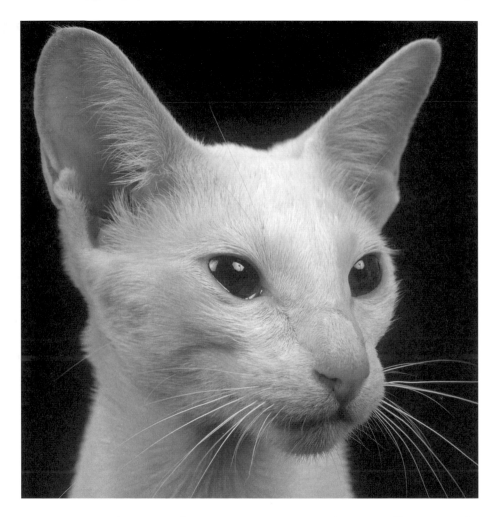

An extreme dieting and exercise campaign might strip off unwanted pounds in a hurry, but the simple fact is that if you can lose it in a week,

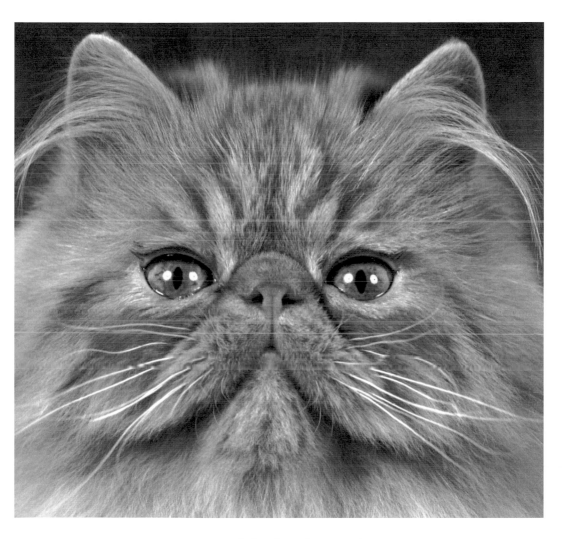

you can put it back on in a week, too.

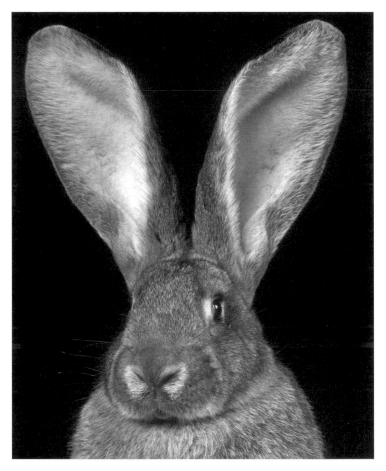

When it comes to effective weight loss, the first and most important step is taking full responsibility for how you look and feel. Your self-belief, integrity, and determination, more than anything else, will determine whether you succeed or fail.

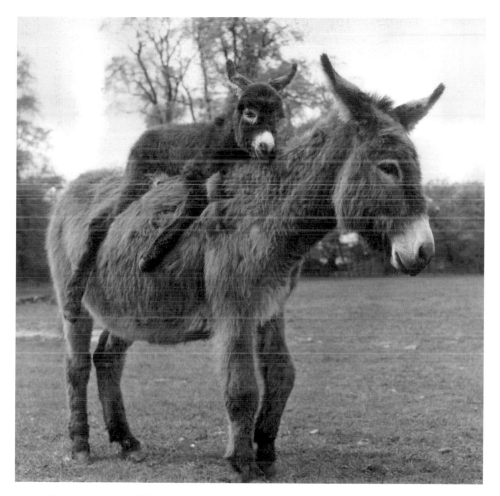

For example, if you are carrying the equivalent of a Cub Scout around your waist, then this is entirely your own doing. Likewise, getting rid of this unwanted burden is up to you and you alone.

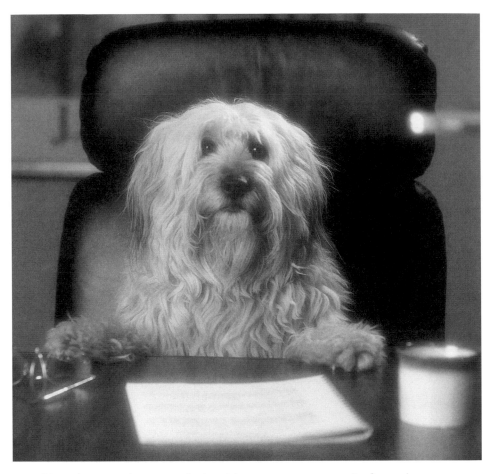

Not that you have to do it without any support. In fact, the very
next step is to see your doctor and get his or her advice.
Listen carefully to what you should and shouldn't do. Remember,
you are losing weight to improve your heath and well-being.

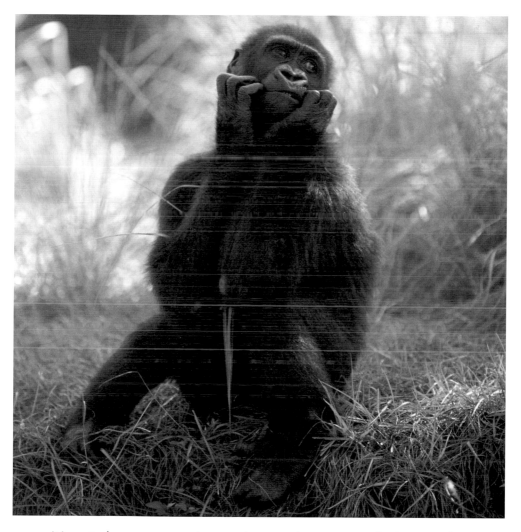

It's not always easy to know where or how to start losing weight.

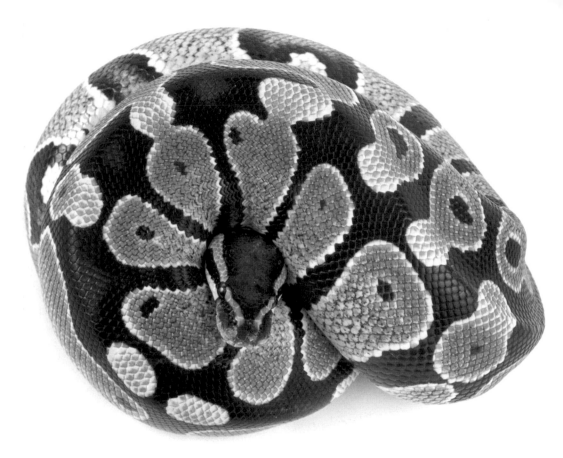

The modern diet and fitness industry is huge and enormously convoluted.
Every single year it squeezes more than $100 billion out of hopeful and
often gullible people. That's more than four times what it cost to put
a man on the moon and, ironically, one hundred times what the
United Nations spends annually on hunger and famine relief.

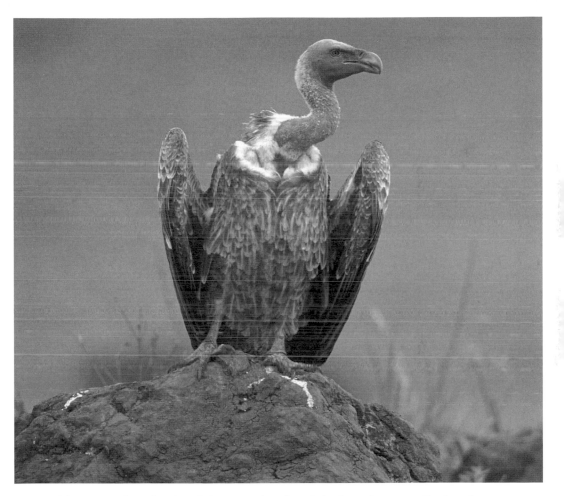

There are hundreds of thousands of weight-loss "experts" who, for a "reasonable" fee, promise to pick the flab from your bones in no time. How can you tell good from bad, worthwhile from worthless?

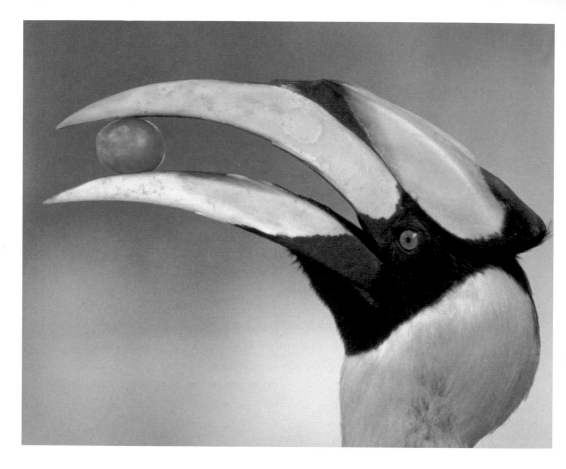

When in doubt, just use your common sense.
There is no such thing as a magic weight-loss pill, and if there
were such a magic pill, no one would ever sell it to you
because then there would be no diet industry.

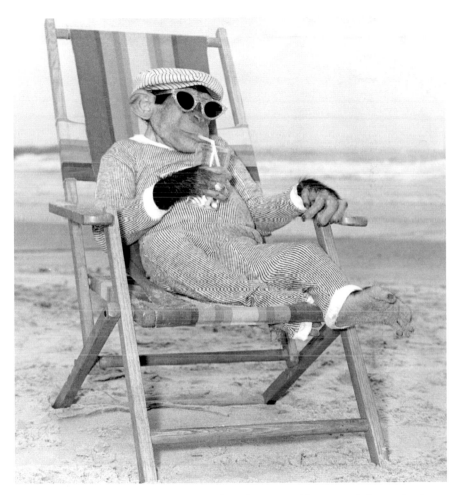

Anything that sounds too good to be true, like a weight-reducing beverage that works wonders even while you continue to live like a lazy slob, probably *is* too good to be true.

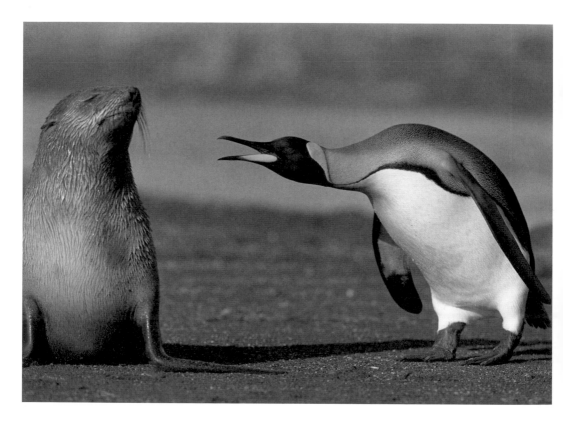

To lose weight you don't need expensive sneakers,
a kooky home gym, or a celebrity personal trainer
who screams at you to do push-ups.

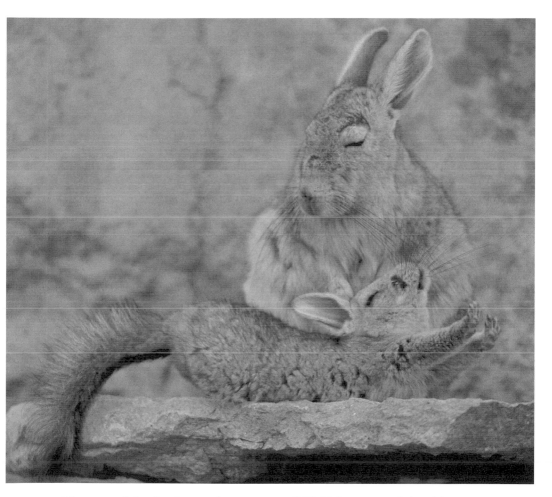

You certainly don't need to go to a $10,000-per-week health spa
to sip celery bouillon and have daily "toning" massages from a
blond, smooth-chested Nordic guy named Sven.

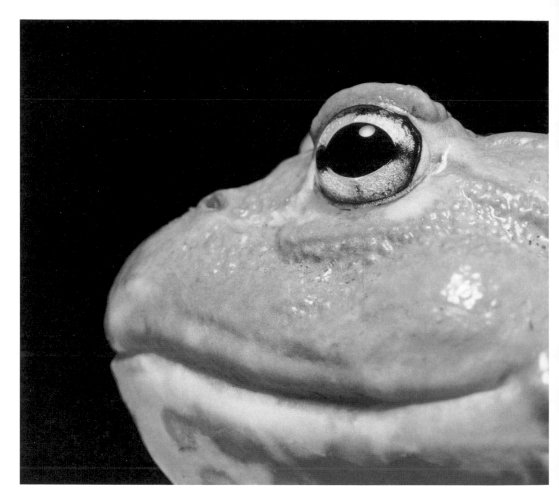

In fact, the good news is that you can relax,
because you already know everything you really need to know
about how to get healthy and lose weight. Everyone does.

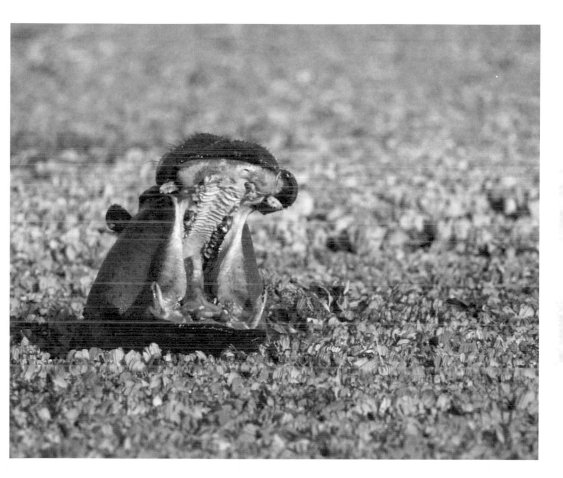

STEP 1: IMPROVE YOUR DIET

It is impossible to think about starting a diet without being
haunted by the unpleasant prospect of drowning in a
bottomless pit of limp leafy greens and bland low-fat dressing.

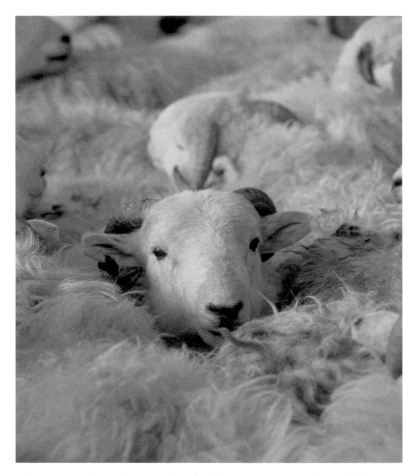

Furthermore, hugely popular fad diets come and go all the time. Many of us have followed the desperate love-handled crowd into the latest dieting craze and then been disappointed because we couldn't achieve or maintain the promised result.

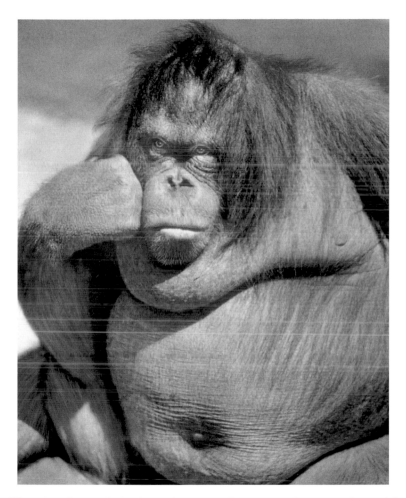

The simple truth is that, despite what some "experts" would
have you believe, improving your diet is not rocket science. It all
boils down to nothing more complicated than *quality* and *quantity*.

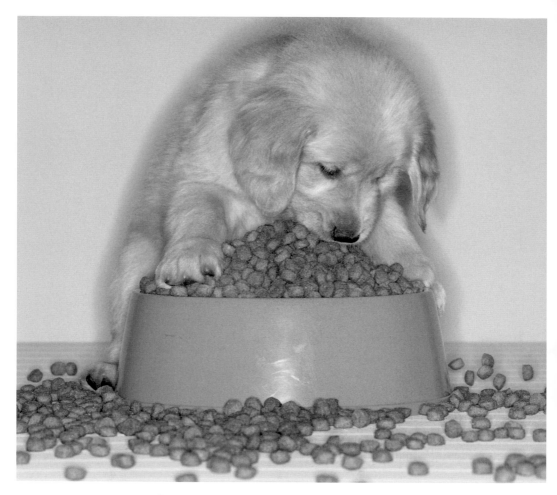

Most of us are eating a lot more than we really need,
and we would all feel much healthier if we reduced
our daily intake considerably.

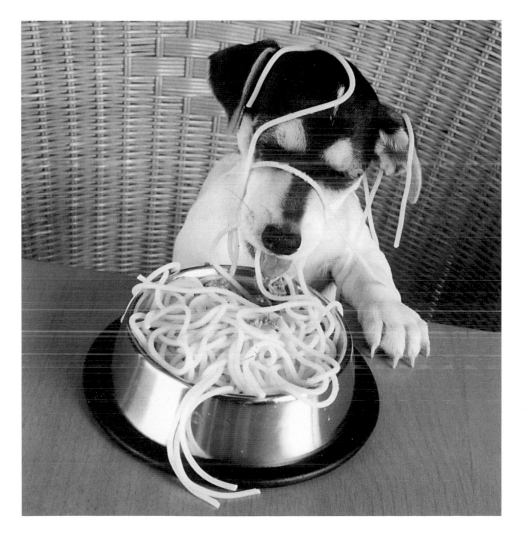

Don't panic! You can still enjoy your favorite meals,

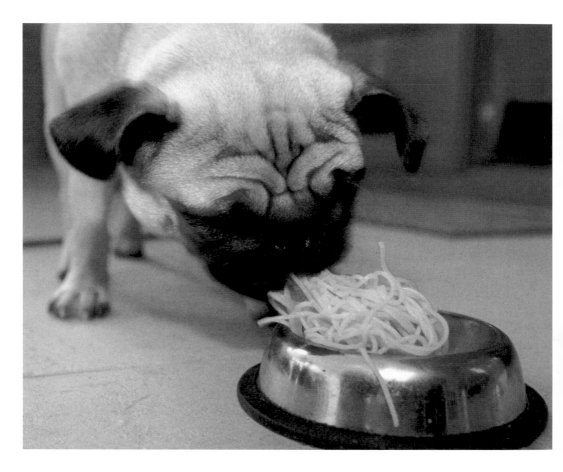

just ease up a little on the portion sizes.

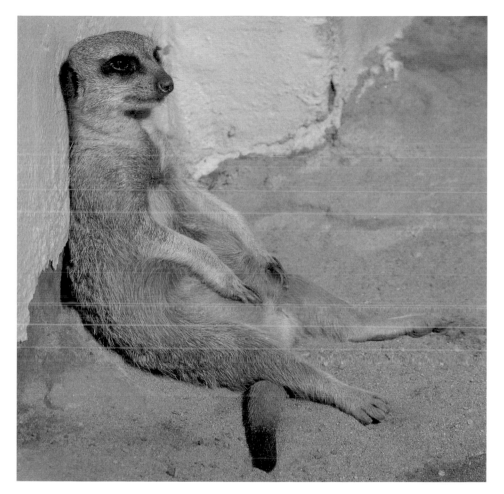

You'll know you've hit the right amount when you really enjoy eating your meal, feel satisfied when you finish, and aren't left with that, "*Ooof*, I need to unbutton the top of my pants or something's going to rupture" feeling.

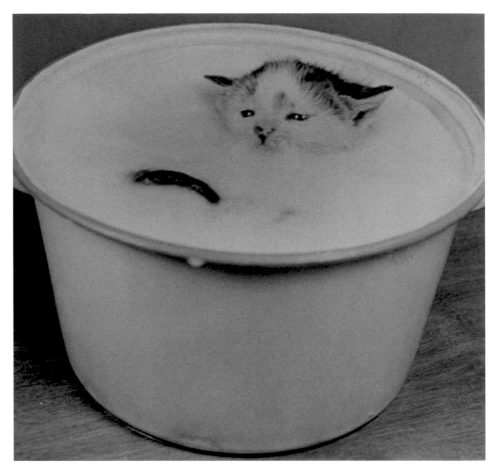

The bigger issue with diet is quality. Many of the processed goods
we buy from the local grocery store and fast-food restaurants
every day have us swimming in unhealthy oils and fats—not to mention
chemical additives such as artificial coloring and flavors—

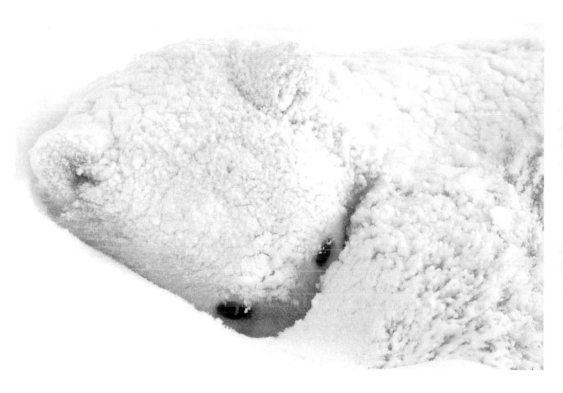

and literally burying ourselves in sugar.

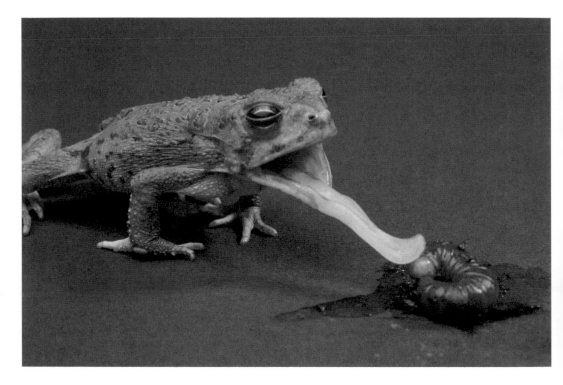

It's enough to make you feel physically sick, or at least run down, irritable, overweight, and generally out of sorts.

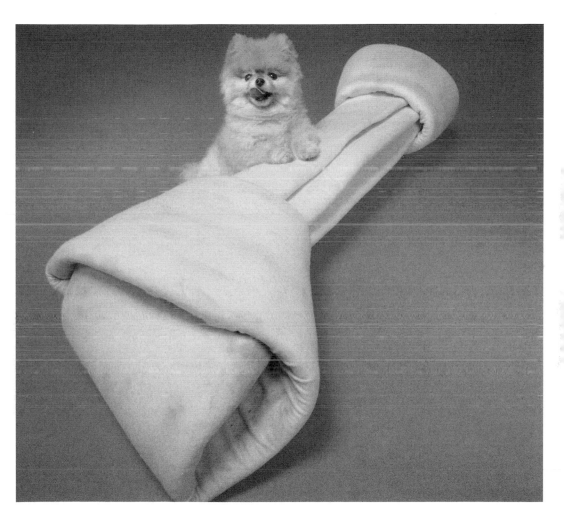

Not that you shouldn't give yourself a treat every now and then.
You really should.

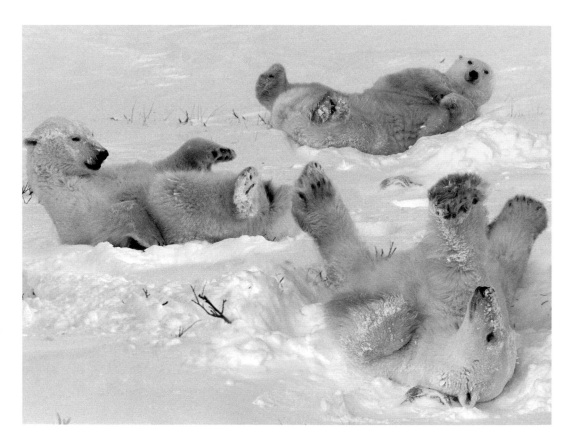

And to forgo the delicious, directionless gluttony of a traditional Thanksgiving feast or Christmas dinner, which leaves everyone bloated and gasping for breath, would be downright unpatriotic!

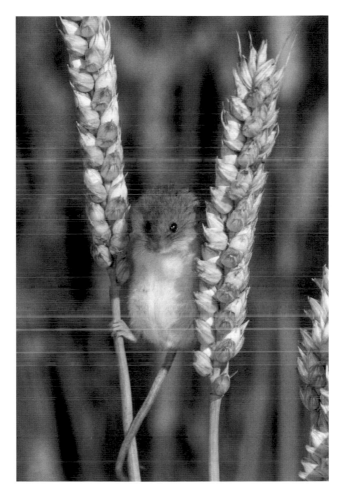

But the rest of the time, if you want to feel great and look your best,
you simply must cut back on the junk food and maintain a
more nutritious, balanced diet with whole grains and cereals,

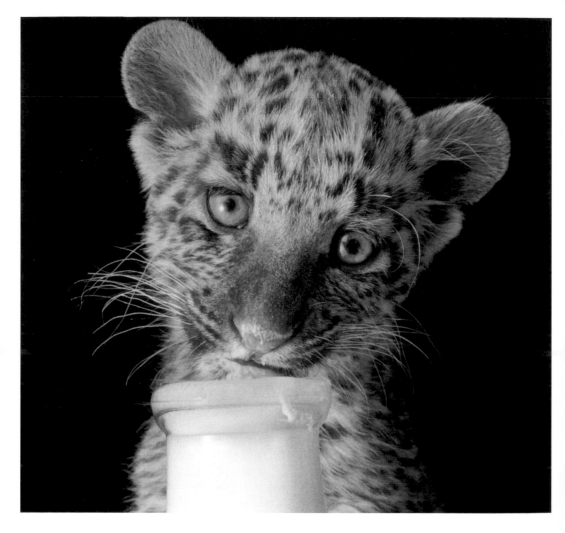

low-fat dairy,

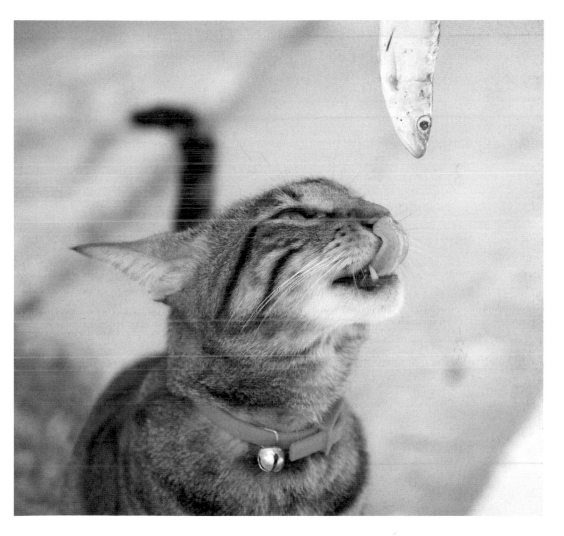

lean protein,

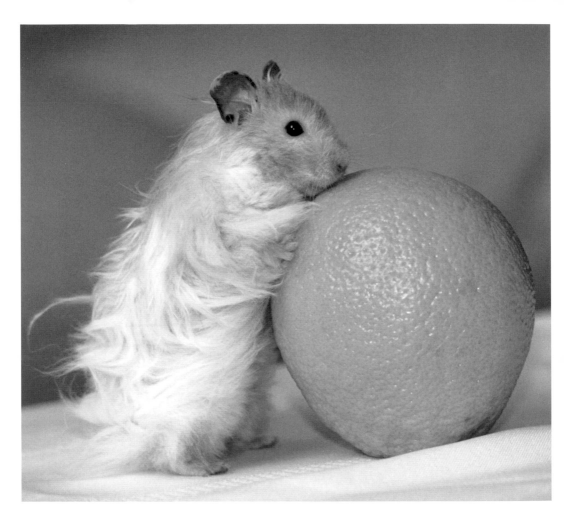

and fresh fruit and vegetables. All of which can be artfully
combined to create every delicious dish you can conceive of.

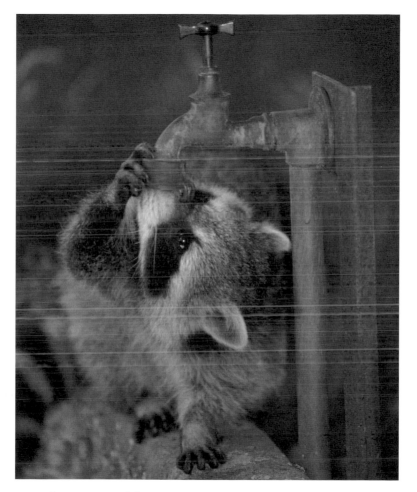

Water is also essential for looking and feeling your best. In fact, truly effective weight loss is impossible without it. The easiest thing you can do to stay healthy is to drink a few extra glasses of water every day.

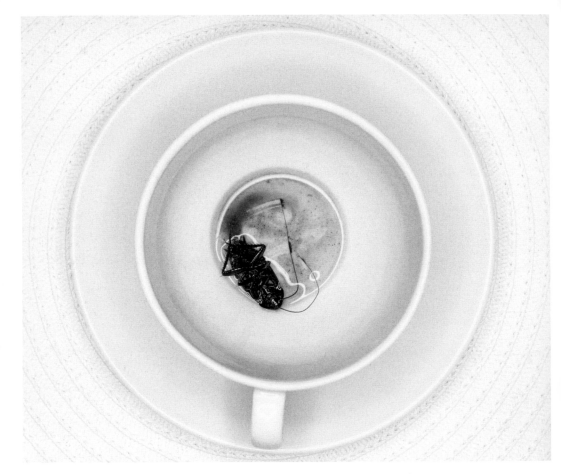

Most of us don't drink nearly enough pure water. To make matters worse, many popular beverages, including alcohol, soda pop, and especially tea and coffee, can actually dehydrate the body. Paradoxically, you are less hydrated after you've finished drinking them than you were before.

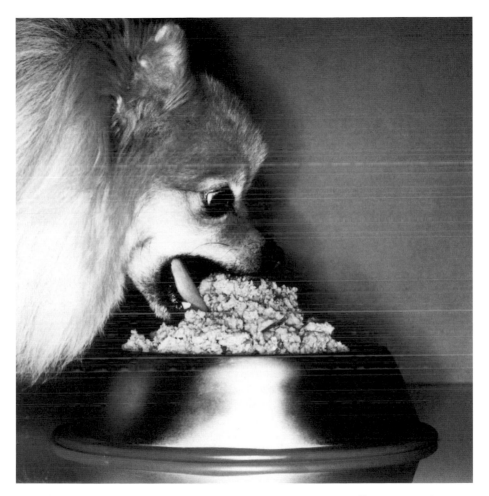

Another simple strategy to lose weight and keep it off is to simply stop shoveling food into your mouth. Most of us need to slow down and enjoy our meals more, rather than treating them like NASCAR refueling stops.

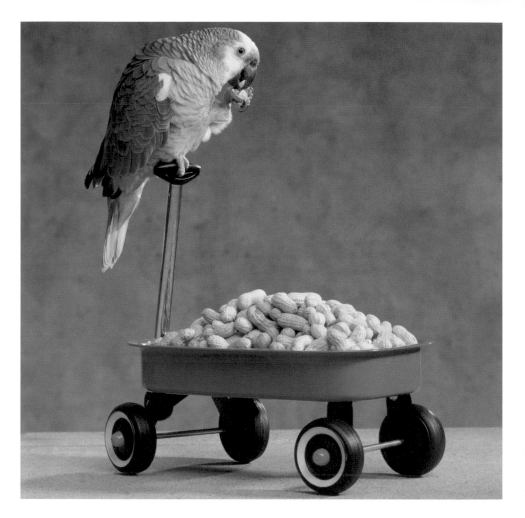

These days most of us are busier than ever, and sometimes eating on the run, unpleasant though it is, cannot be avoided.

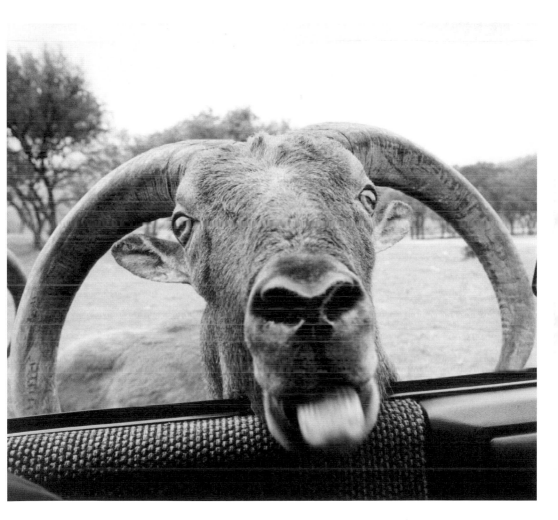

But as we've all learned, nothing wonderful or life-changing
ever came out of a drive-through service window.

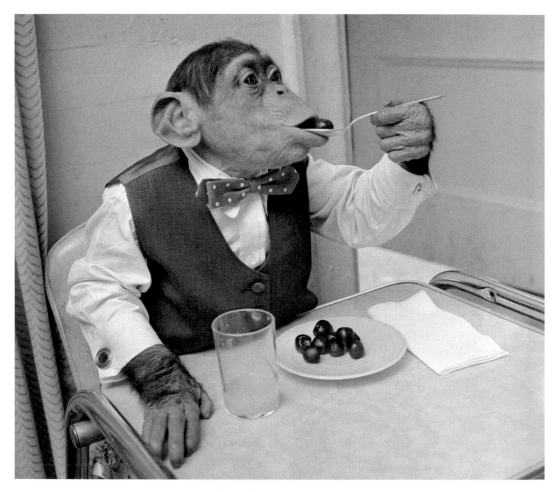

So remember, it will really make a huge difference in your
quality of life and especially your health and well-being
if you just stop and enjoy what you are eating.

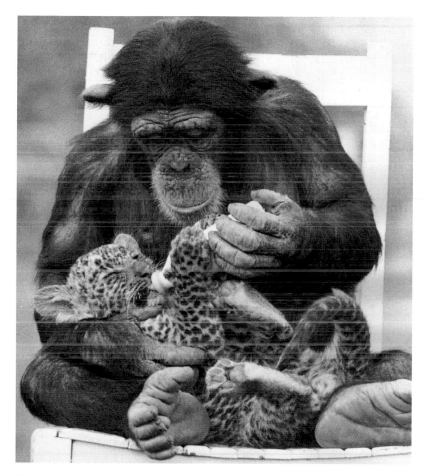

The fundamental principle of improving your diet comes down to this:
There was once a time in your life when all your nutritional needs
were met without your having to lift a finger.
Well, those days are obviously long gone.

59

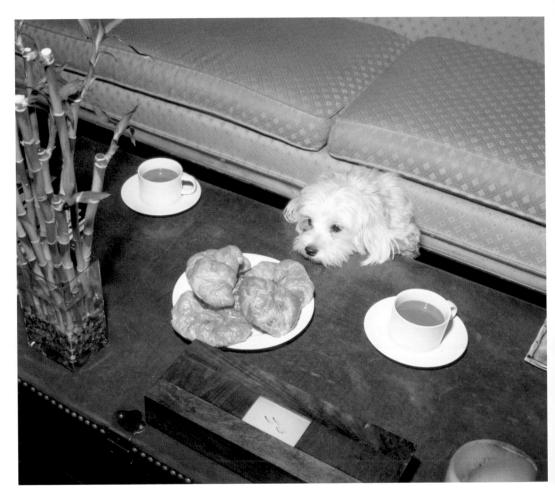

Now it's all up to you and the many small but ultimately profound choices you make each and every day. "Do I really need to eat another pastry with my coffee?"

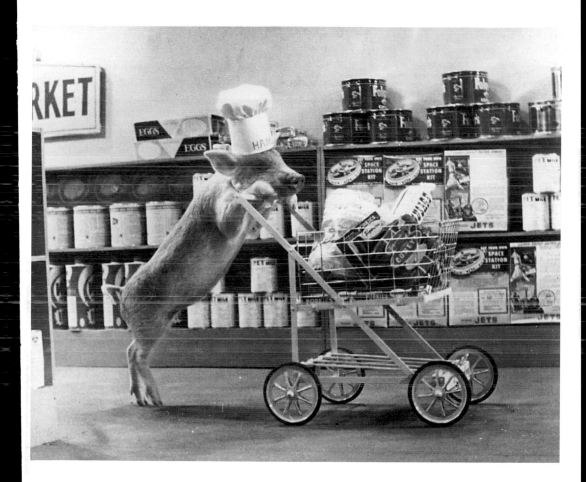

These are the choices that form the bedrock of all your dietary habits.
The decisions you make at the supermarket

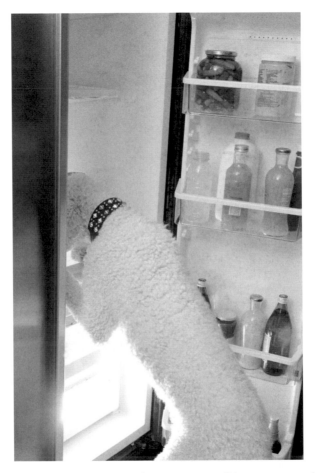

dictate the decisions you make at your refrigerator, and so on.
By making the best choices from the beginning, you massively increase
your chances of success. The key is making it easier and more
enjoyable to eat well. It's really that simple.

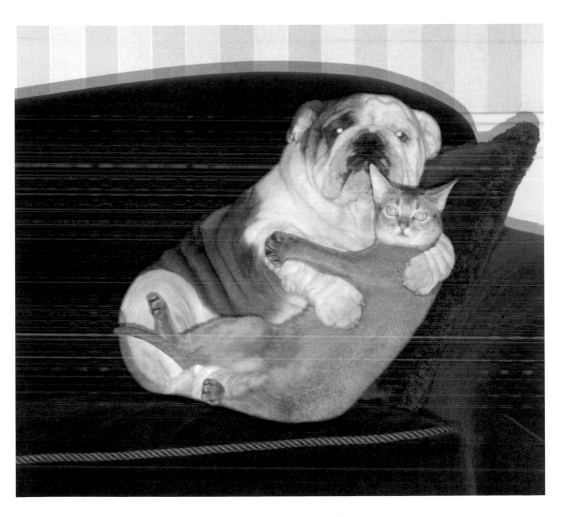

STEP 2: DO A LITTLE MORE EXERCISE

Nothing terrifies long-term couch potatoes like the threat of exercise.

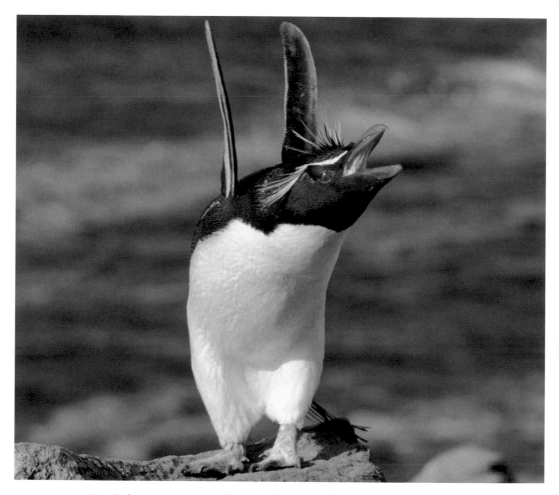

Such fears are not unfounded. Since the invention of Lycra,
exercise has built up a deservedly unpleasant reputation,
thanks to psychotic aerobics instructors,

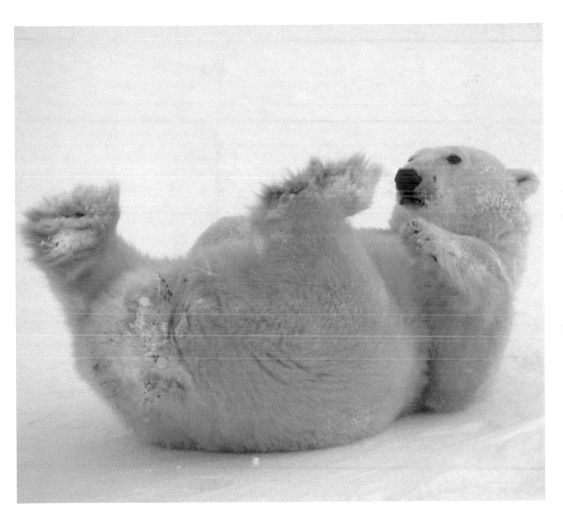

mind-numbingly boring and repetitive workouts
featuring wholly undignified ab exercises,

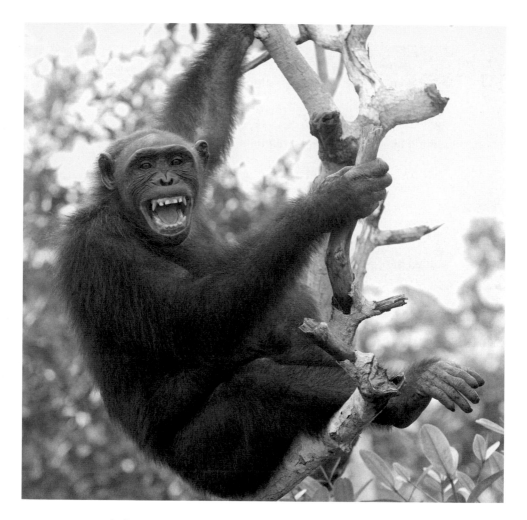

and the sweat-soaked, grunting cacophony of painful,
unnecessarily complex gym equipment.

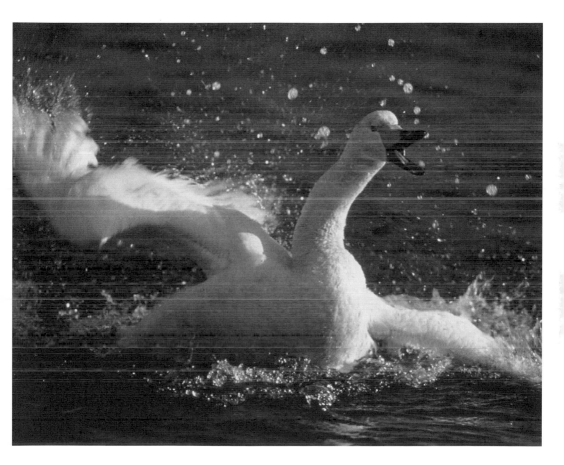

But it doesn't have to be like that. To get into great shape
you don't have to swim the English Channel

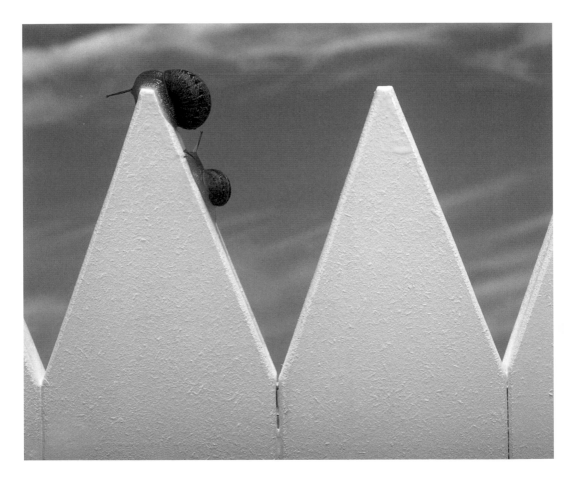

or grind your way through the Tour de France.

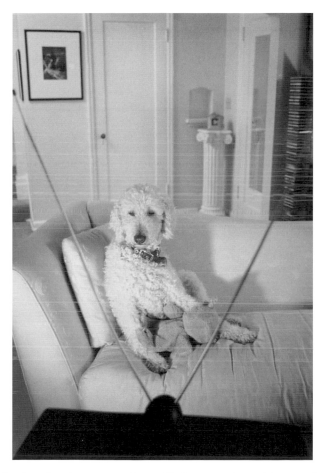

Exercise is simply about getting off the couch and becoming active.
That will be the toughest step. But if you can turn off the TV,
put down the newspaper, and walk out the door, you are already
well on your way to better health and a better body.

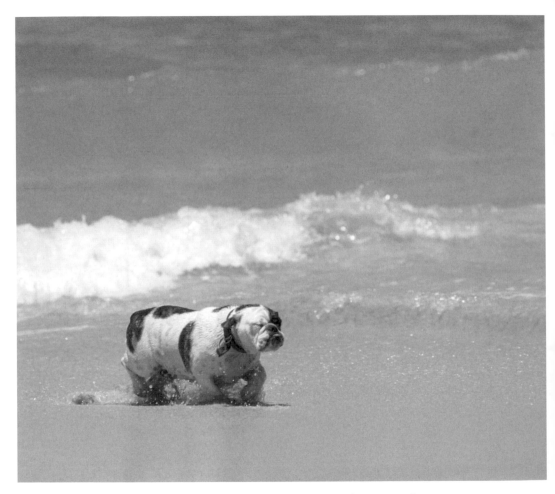

I'm not saying it will be easy. It won't be. Your first run
along the beach isn't going to look anything like
the opening scenes of *Baywatch*,

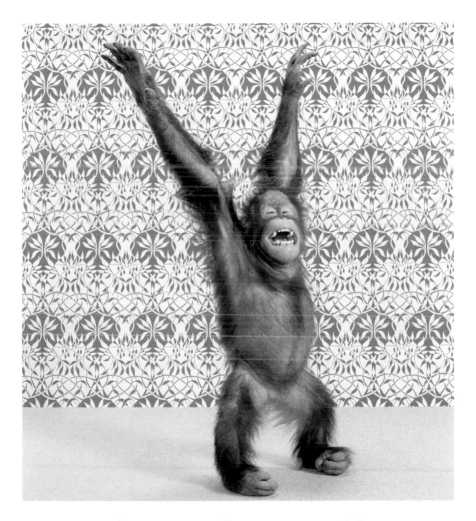

and you may soon discover some sore joints
and stiff muscles you never knew you had.

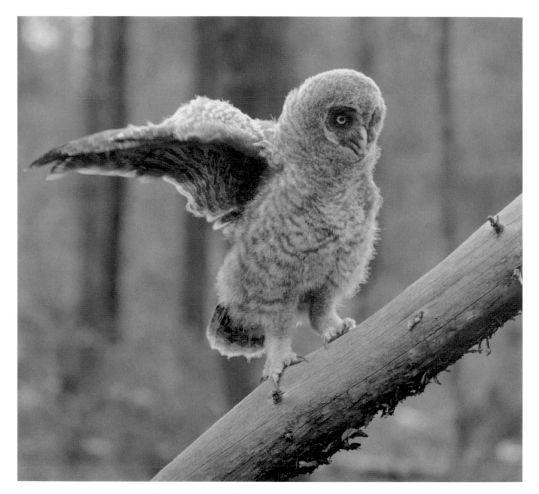

Just stick with it and gradually increase your level of intensity.
Soon you'll start losing weight while increasing your strength and fitness,
and you'll be surprised at just how much more energy you have.

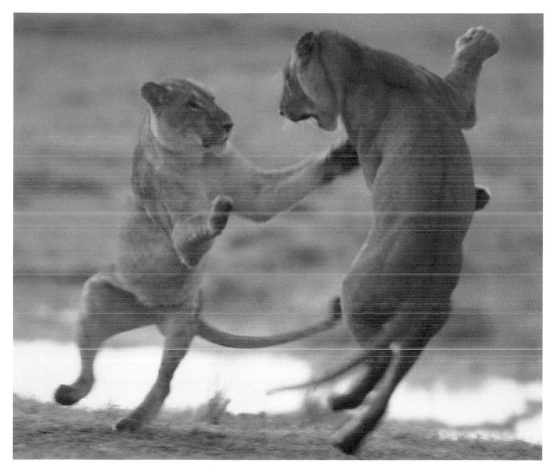

You don't need to be stuck on a treadmill in a smelly gym.
There is a whole world of weird and wonderful activities for you to
enjoy while you get your heart pumping. For example, a friendly game
of touch football can be both a terrific workout and a social event. 73

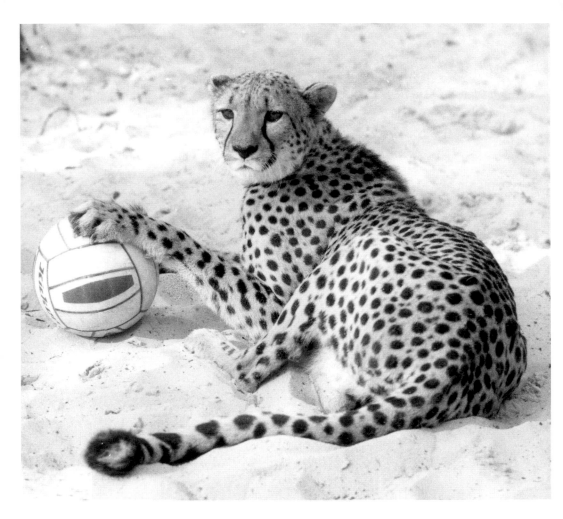

Beach volleyball is a fun way to work up a sweat
before stretching out in the sunshine to improve your tan,

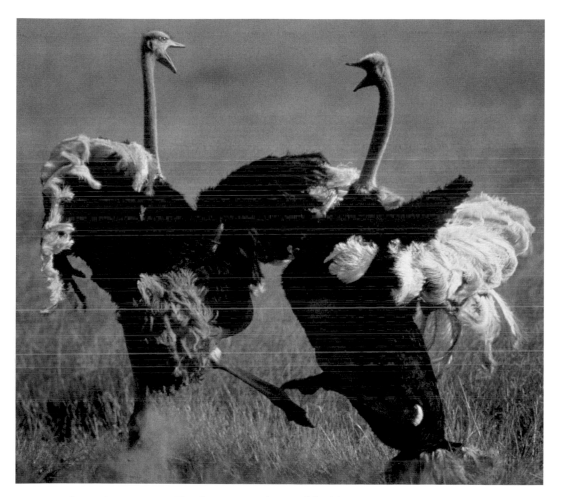

and combat sports like karate, judo, and kickboxing are an exciting way
to build self-confidence and burn calories. Frankly, after a tough day
it just feels really good to beat the living daylights out of somebody.

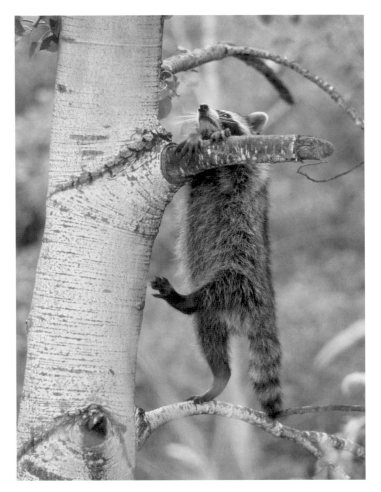

With imagination and effort you can turn virtually any fun activity into quality exercise. Even tossing a Frisbee around can be a surprisingly tough workout, especially if you play near tall trees and your aim is lousy.

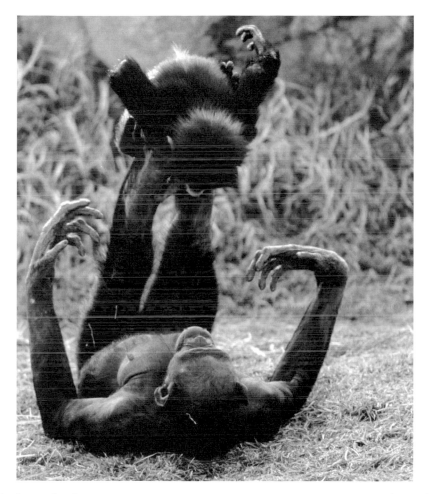

In fact, the best way to increase your exercise is to get outside and have more fun with your family and friends. After all, isn't that one of the biggest reasons to get healthy and energized in the first place?

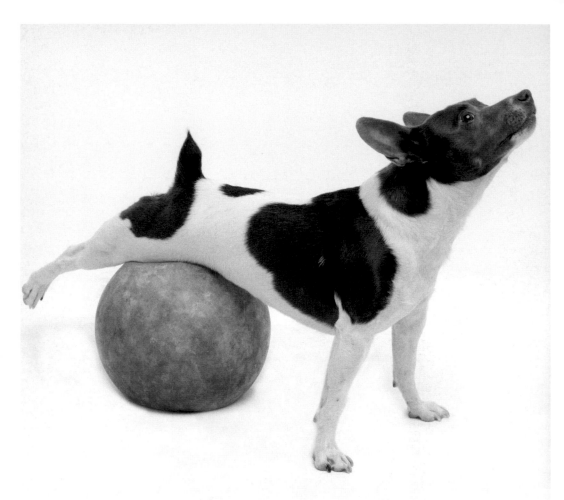

Just about everyone will have a time when their exercise regimen loses momentum for one reason or another.

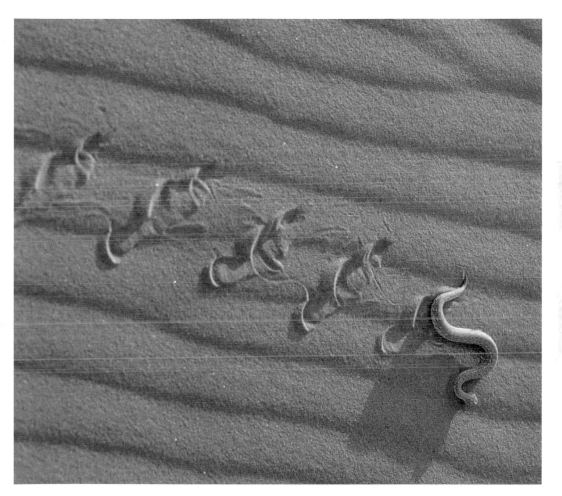

"I'll catch cold," "I'm too busy," "It's raining," "It's the final episode of *Survivor* tonight." It's oh so easy to come up with more and more excuses to keep wriggling out of your exercise commitments again and again.

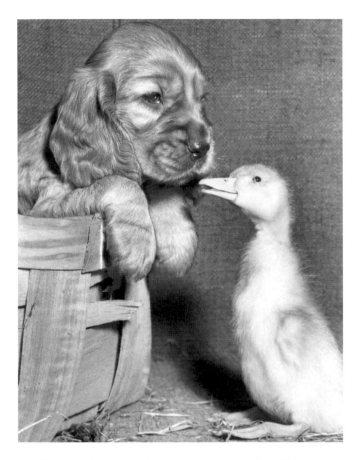

To prevent stalling, it helps to have an exercise buddy—an active friend you don't want to let down by not turning up on time or not giving your best effort. It might be a pal you meet for a walk instead of a cup of coffee, someone who is likely to pop by and ask, "Who's up for a game of tennis?" instead of flopping in front of the TV.

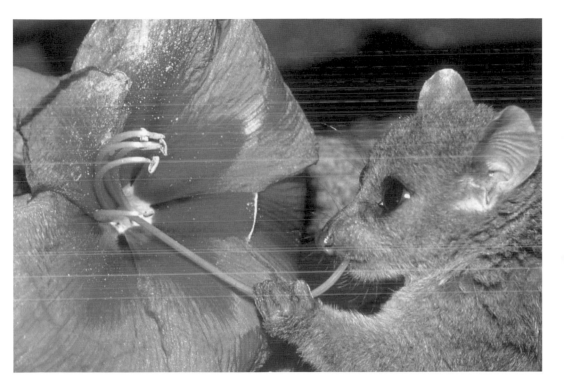

If you are tired, your motivation is weak, and you would rather
be on your own, just sit down for ten minutes to catch your breath
and eat a piece of fruit or have a sports energy drink.

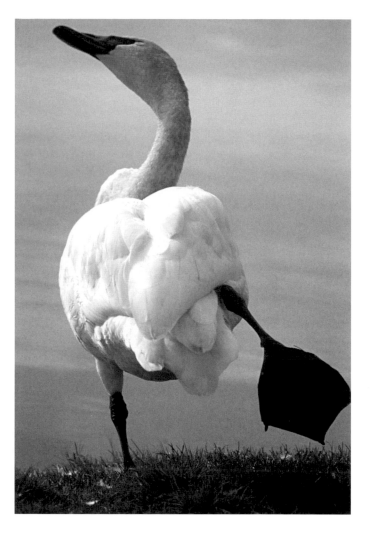

Then start moving! Even a slow sunset stroll will do.

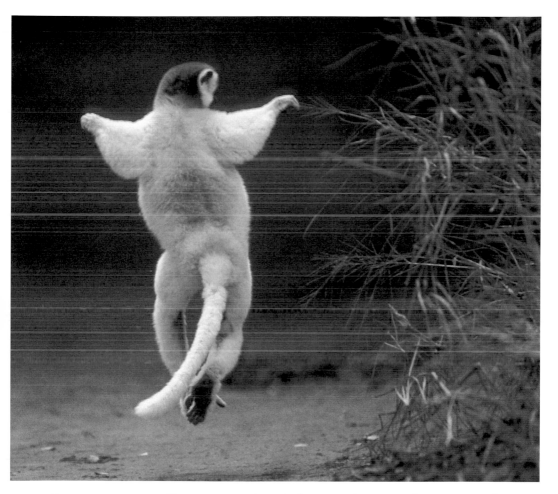

Pretty soon you will start to revive. Before you know it, the spring will
be back in your step and your fatigue and pudgy past will be further and
further behind you. That's the power and the purpose of exercise.

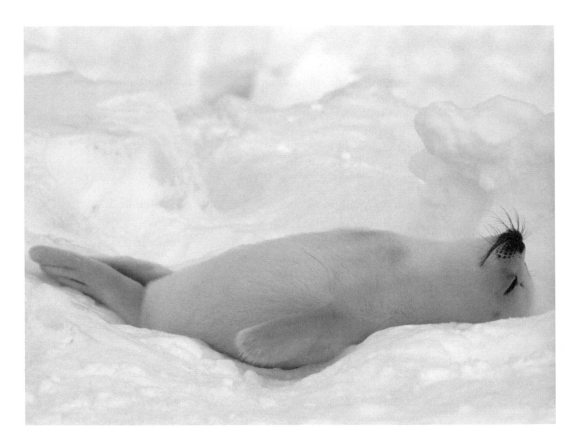

<u>STEP 3: GET SOME REST</u>

The last piece of the health-plan puzzle is by far the easiest
to acquire, but it is the one that most people miss, and that's why
they subsequently fail to lose weight. They just need to get
enough rest every day, especially a proper night's sleep.

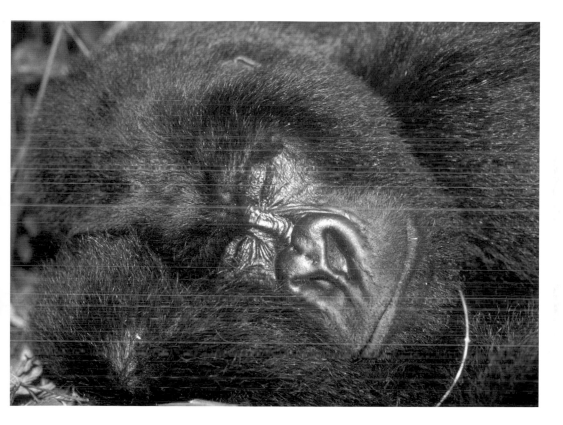

Life really is an endurance sport, and getting your eight hours of
quality sleep every night is essential to recharge your batteries,
repair tired muscles, and keep your immune system working well.
This is especially true when you start an exercise plan or change your diet.
In fact, you may even need a little more sleep than usual.

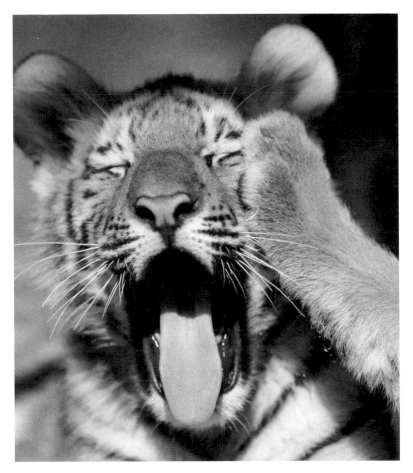

When your body needs a rest and you refuse to take it,
the wheels starting falling off pretty quickly. One of the first symptoms
of fatigue is that you will lose the desire to exercise properly,
and you will be less inclined to eat well.

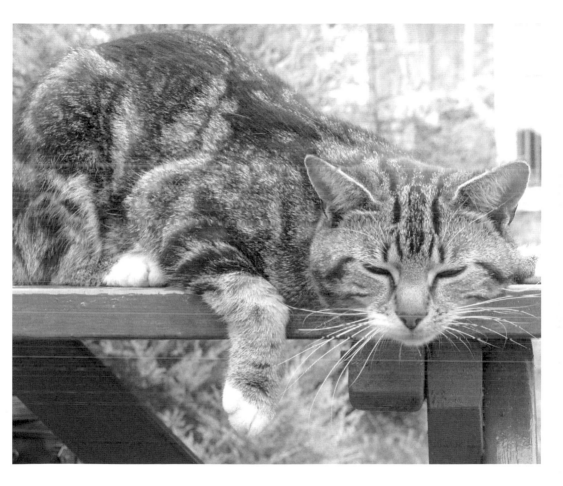

In simple terms:
Busy people who don't rest properly become tired people.

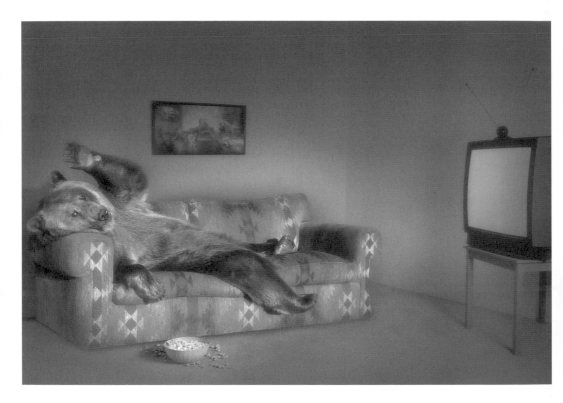

Tired people who don't rest properly become lazy people.

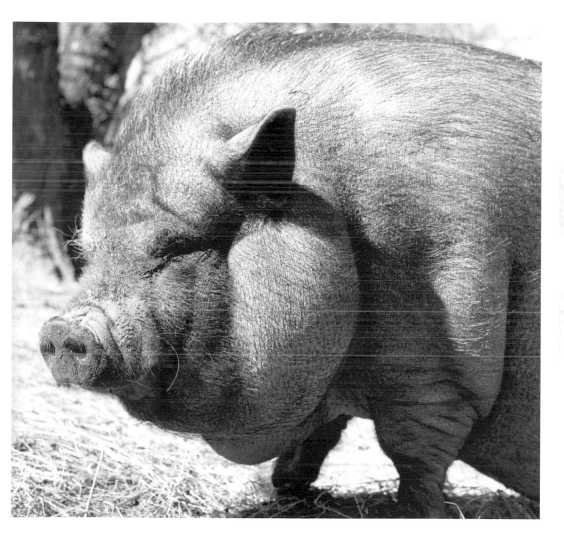

And lazy people become fat people.

89

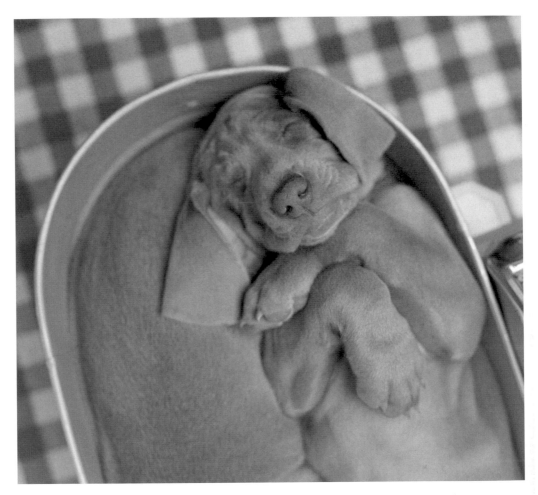

If you don't rest properly, your health and your weight-loss plans are guaranteed to fail. By sleeping soundly each night you will get fitter and healthier much faster and stay that way longer.

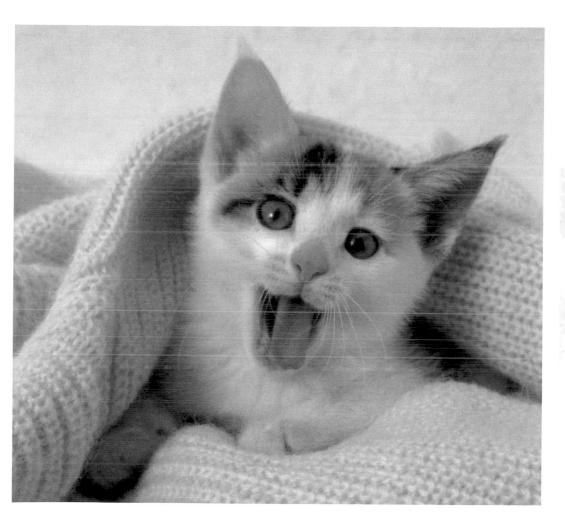

Best of all, you'll wake up refreshed every day, capable of getting
the most out of life because you'll feel ready to take on the world.

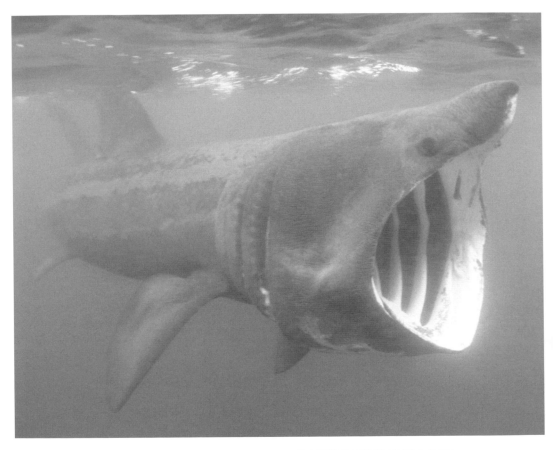

THE GOLDEN RULES OF EFFECTIVE WEIGHT LOSS

The first golden rule is simply to keep your big mouth shut.
This immediately reduces your intake of excessive calories and
stops you from driving people crazy by going on and on
about your diet and regaining your ideal weight.

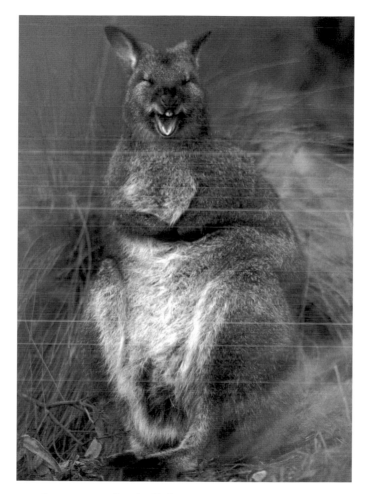

"So anyway, I power-walked all the way to the corner store today, and yesterday I ate nothing but sunflower seeds and asparagus. I'm right on track to be a size four in time for my niece's bat mitzvah!"

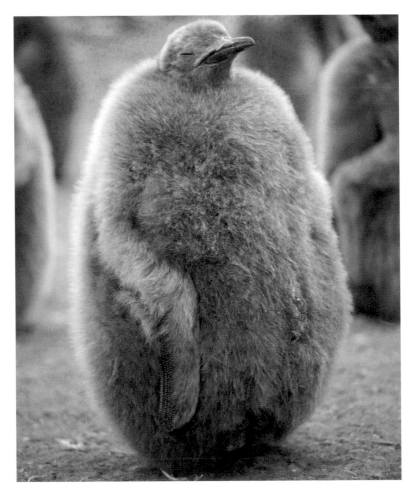

It's far better to maintain a dignified silence
throughout every stage of your campaign—say less, do more.
After all, your weight loss is no one else's business.

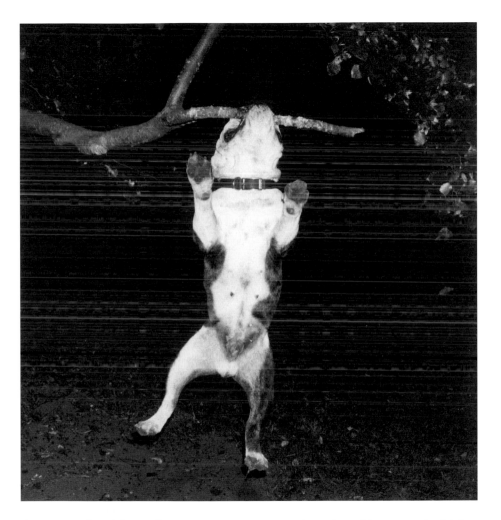

The second golden rule is to maintain your discipline. You must hold fast
to your weight-loss goals one day at a time. *Do not quit on yourself!*

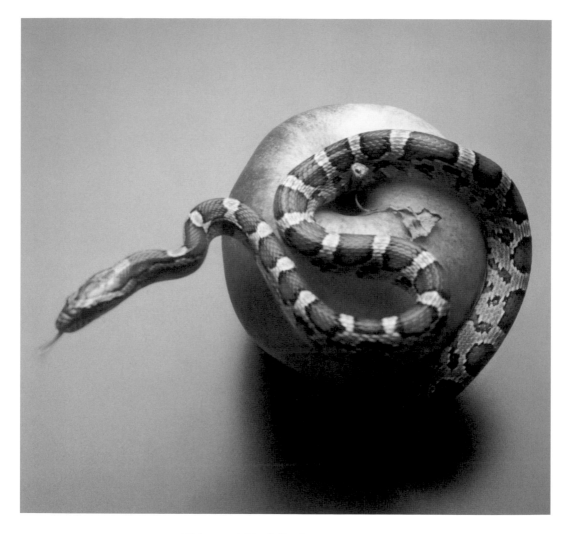

This world is full of temptations.

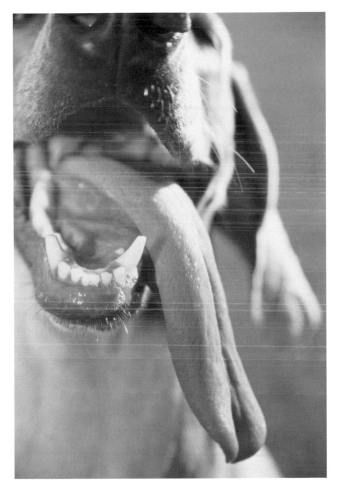

You might see an ad on TV for spicy buffalo wings or catch
an intoxicating whiff of fresh-baked cookies or a BBQ grill heating up,
and the evil little voices begin,

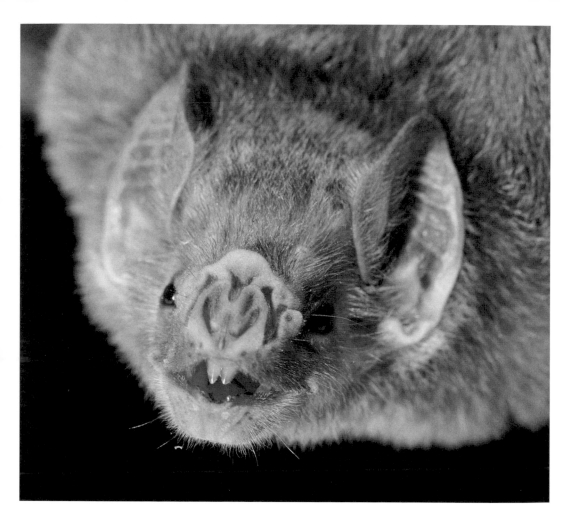

"Eeaaaaaat the burgerrr, tryyyyyyy the mud caaake,
just unwrap one leeeeetle chocolaaate."

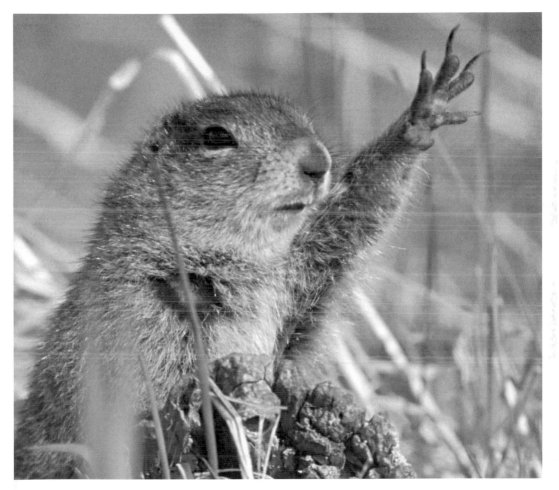

If unchecked, these voices will increase until you feel sick with longing and stupefied by your cravings. In extreme cases dazed victims actually start reaching for imaginary candy bars and phantom pizza slices.

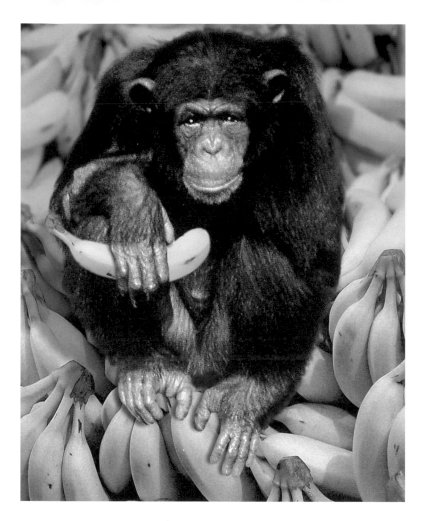

You may just start with a teeny-weeny taste, just one bite,
just enough to get the flavor on your taste buds,

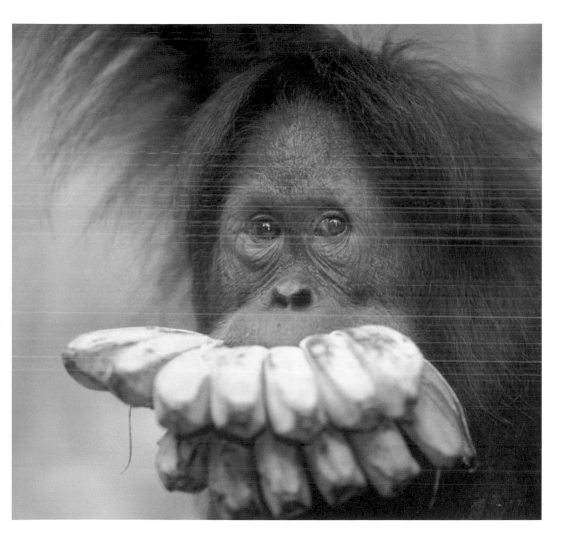

but one thing leads to another, and soon things get out of control.

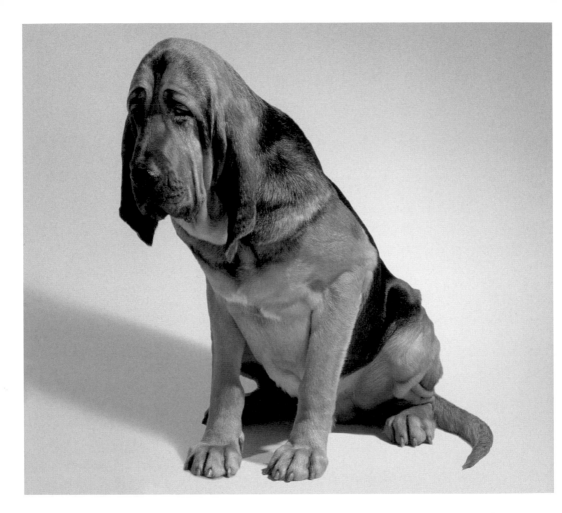

It's only when the feeding frenzy has subsided that the damage hits home.
I assure you, regret wears size XXXXXXL pants.

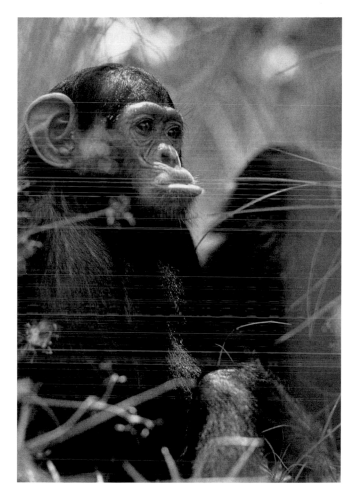

If you hit a weak spot, the best thing to do is take a walk and think about your goals and what they mean to you. You could also talk to someone close, especially an exercise buddy, if you think you need help.

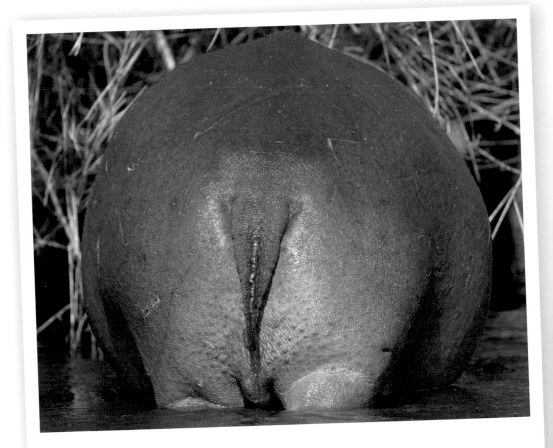

If that doesn't work, take out your old "fat photos"
from last summer and remind yourself what is at stake.

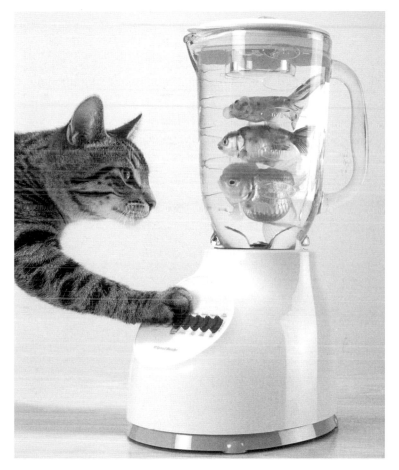

Remember, "An empty stomach is the devil's deli." Whip up a low-calorie snack at home and drink a glass or two of water to ease your hunger pangs. Do whatever you must to keep moving in the right direction.

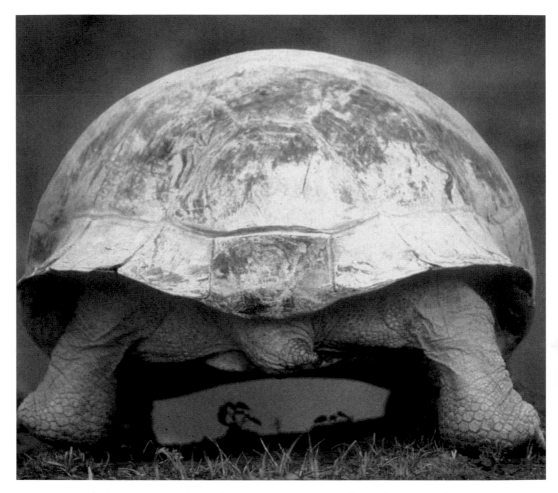

Real discipline is about keeping things simple and staying focused on what really matters. All you have to do is maintain a healthy consistency and move toward your goals gradually but relentlessly.

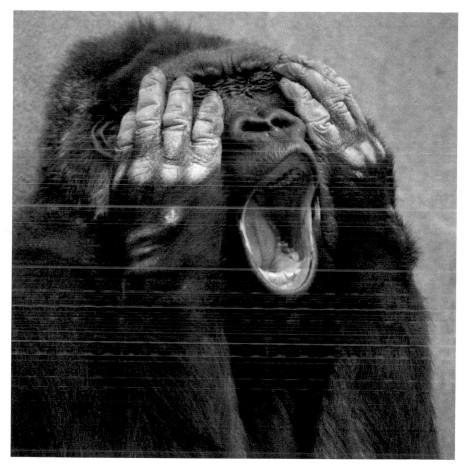

Don't let your diet and exercise plan take over your life
so you completely lose touch with the real world. "Oh my God, I just
ate a grain of sugar! I must punish myself by repeatedly
slamming my head in the refrigerator door!"

107

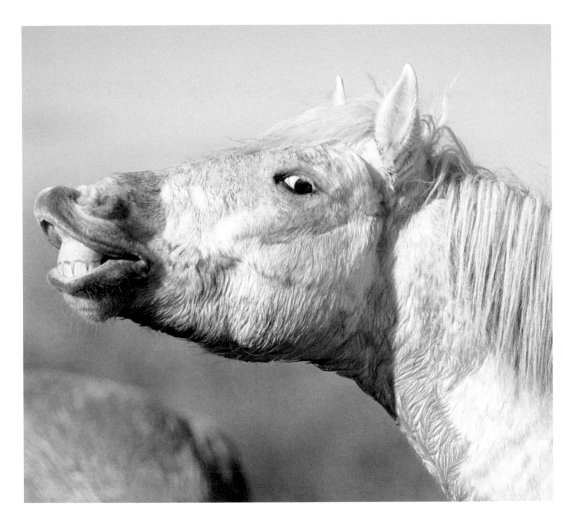

The last golden rule, perhaps the most important of them all,
is to be patient and positive.

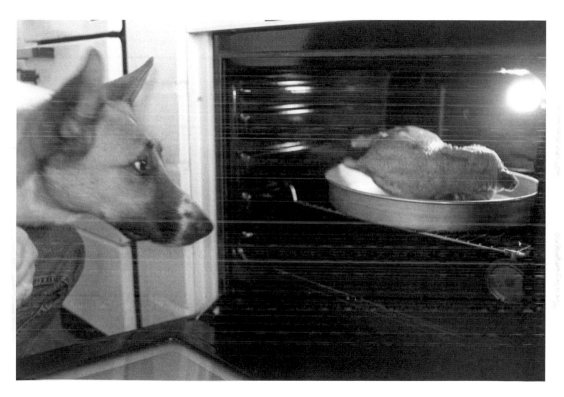

There is no secret, super-duper short cut to effective
long-term health and weight loss. Most good things in life
take time and are worth waiting for.

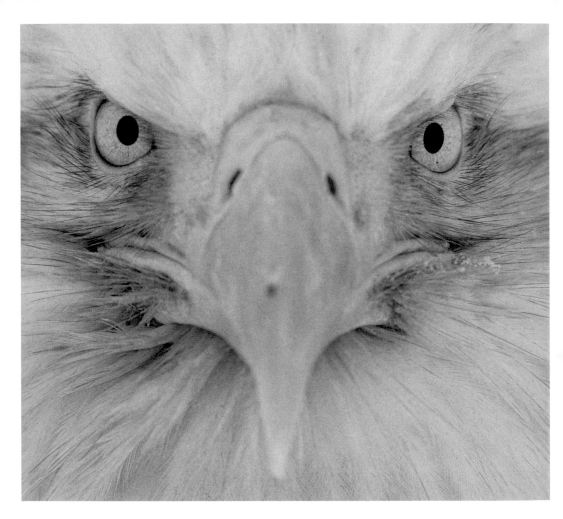

Not every day will be jam-packed with giggles and candy canes.
You will probably feel hungry and cranky every now and then,

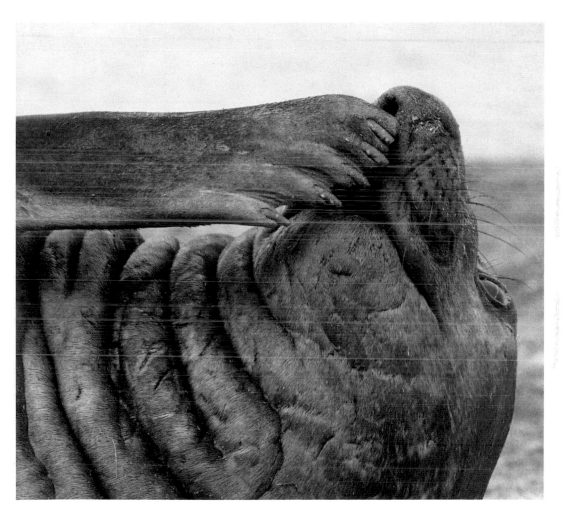

and you might find your tummy takes a while
to adjust to your new diet.

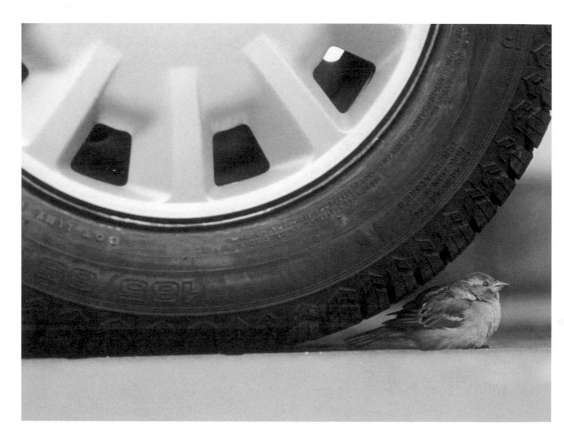

You may feel depressed because nothing seems to be happening, and on your worst days, you might wish all your troubles could be swept away for good.

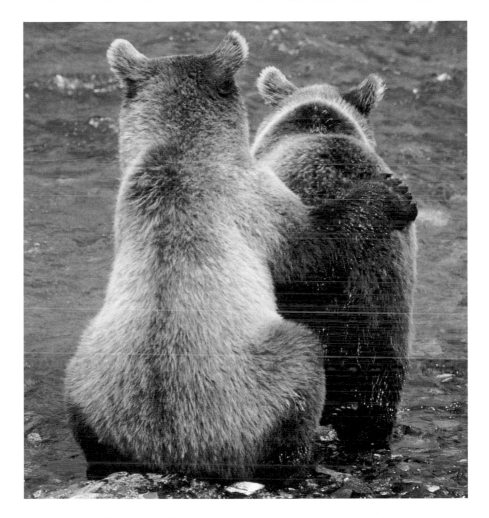

It's likely you'll need a shoulder to cry on or at least
a few words of encouragement every once in a while.

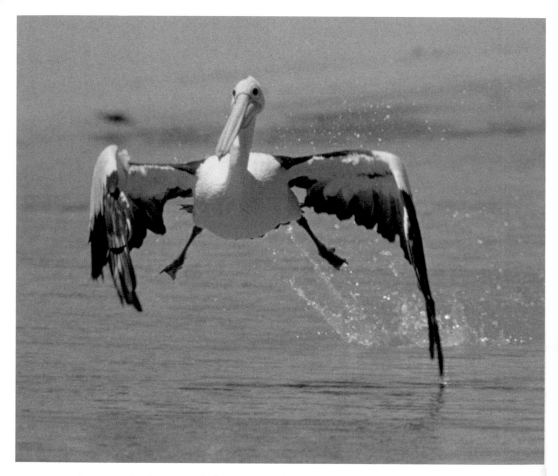

Just remind yourself that every day you continue means you are one day closer to achieving your goal of looking and feeling great. It may take a little while to get your dream off the ground, but if you follow the golden rules, you *will* get there. It's guaranteed.

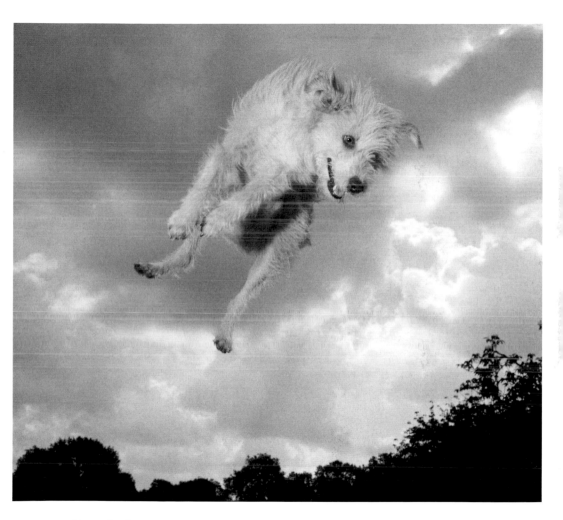

Even before you lose much weight, you may notice that you are thinking more clearly, feeling fresher, and have a *lot* more energy. 115

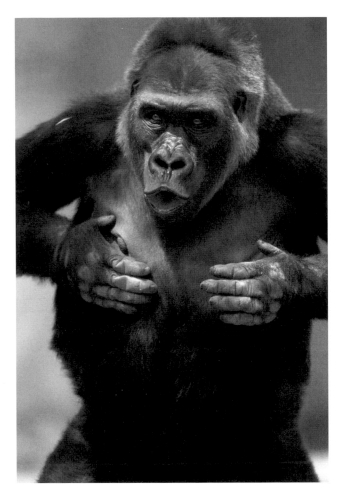

Then one day you'll be in a dressing room trying on something, and you'll notice exciting changes. Maybe your tummy looks flatter, or your love handles are vanishing, or your thighs look more toned.

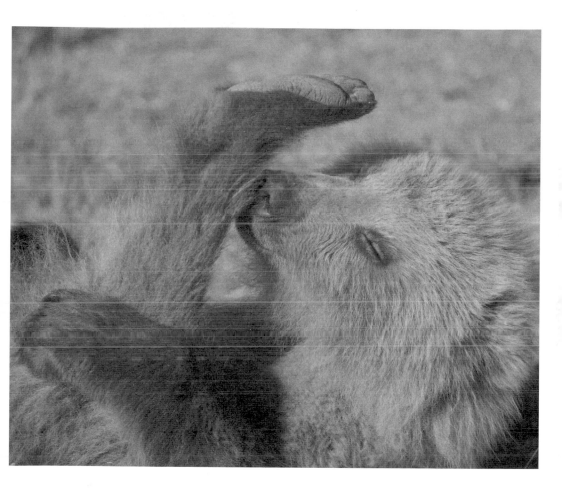

Pretty soon you will start falling in love
with a whole new you.

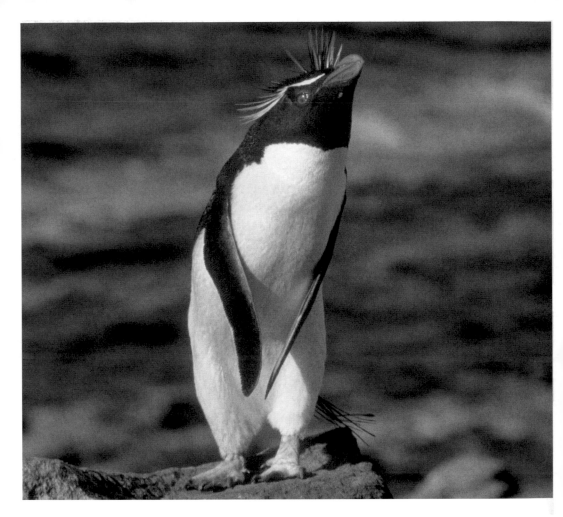

You'll feel full of life, slim and strong, happy and healthy, and, dare I say, oh sooo sexy!

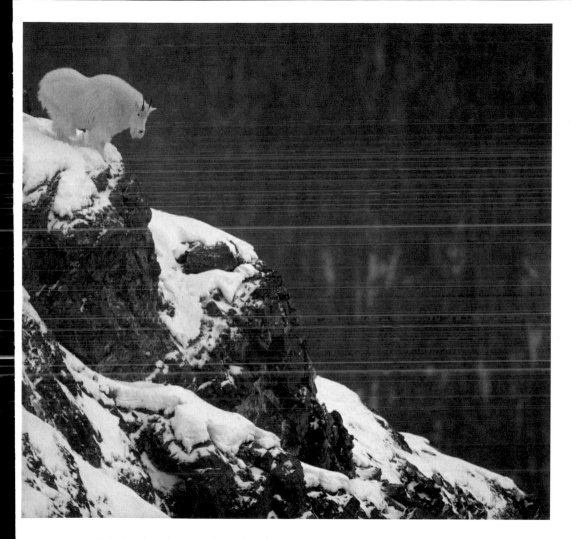

This is the time to look back on just how far you have come,

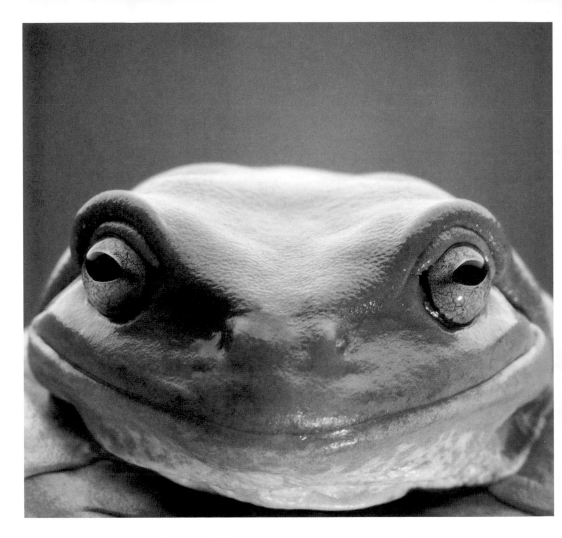

and that will be a very, very good day indeed.

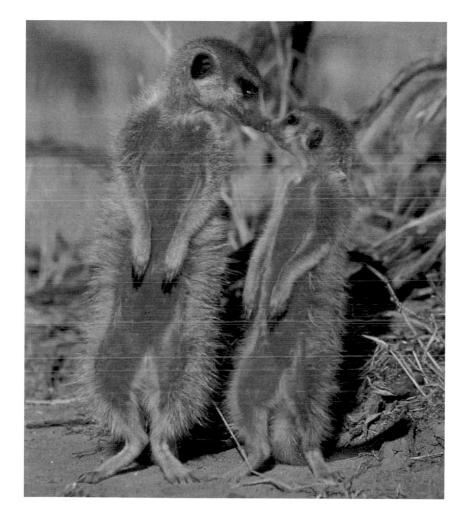

Your newfound magnetism will have an immediate and overwhelming
effect on everybody you meet whether you like it or not.

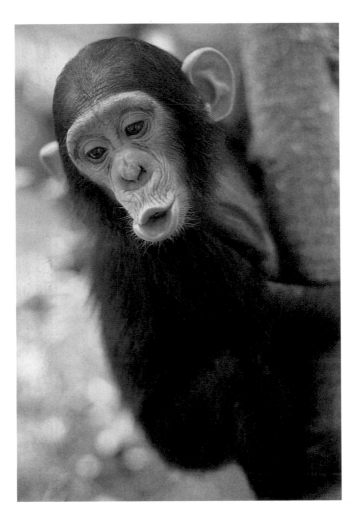

On the street, people will shamelessly wolf whistle
when you stroll by,

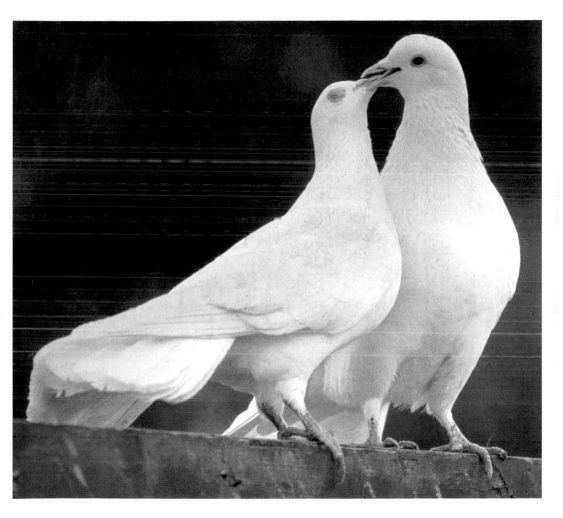

gorgeous strangers may walk right up and kiss you on the mouth,
just like V-J Day in Times Square,

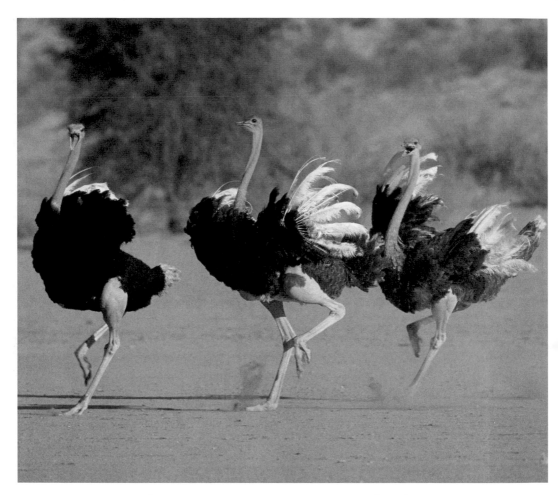

and irritating "jogger types" in tiny nylon shorts
and experimental sneakers will constantly plead with you
to go running with them.

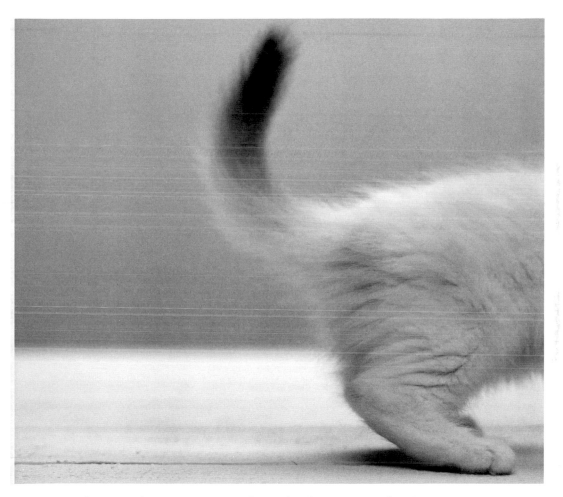

As your diet improves and weight decreases, other important
appetites will increase. At parties you will become aware
of people admiring your firm and shapely caboose,

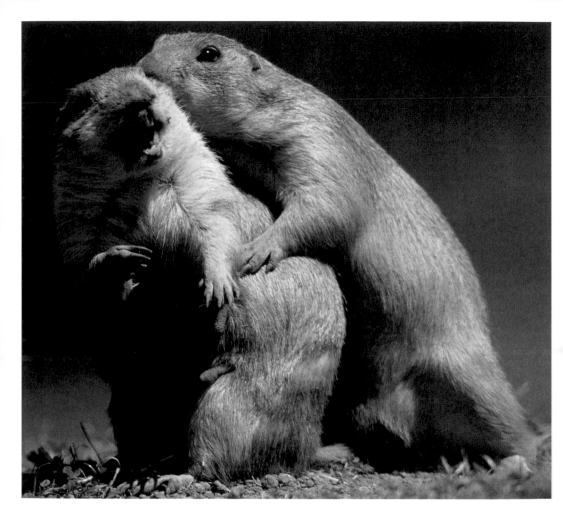

and when you get home your beloved simply won't be able
to keep their love-hungry hands off your sensuously sculpted body.

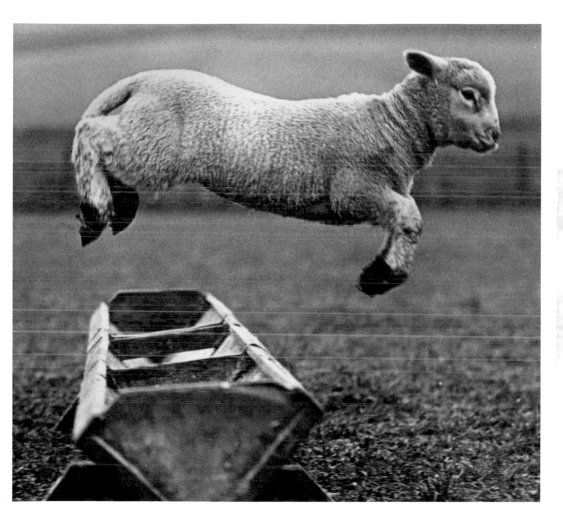

Having effectively harnessed all your passion, self-belief, and discipline to overcome such a huge life hurdle, you may well become unstoppable.

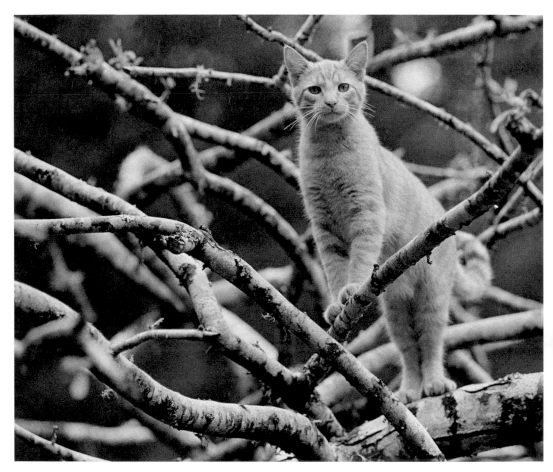

You'll probably go on to apply what you have learned about yourself
to confront your worst fears and achieve your greatest dreams.
But then, you'll face the enormous challenge of what to do
with all your extra free time.

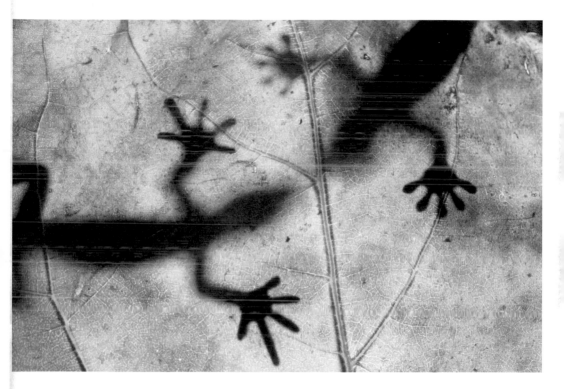

As if that wasn't tough enough, when you realize that someone
who substantially reduces their silhouette can enjoy
a much larger life with bigger sunsets and broader horizons,

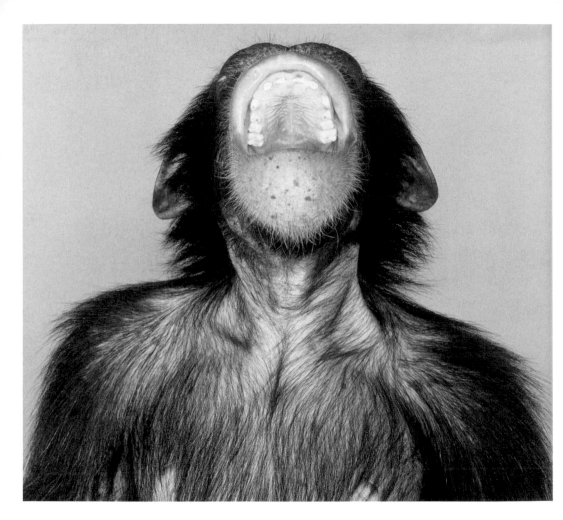

not to mention a greatly increased lung capacity
for laughing louder and longer,

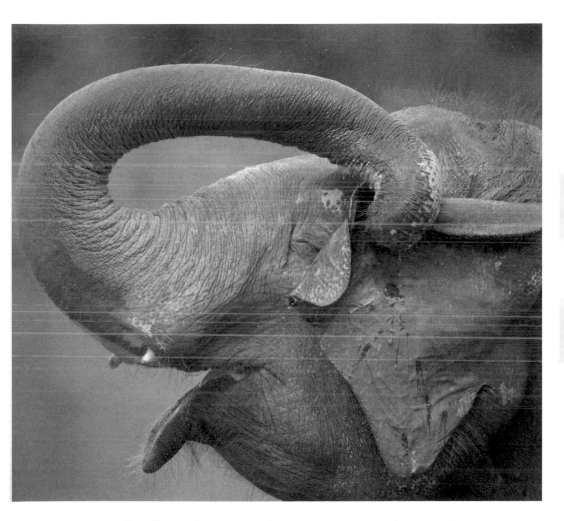

you may well pull your hair out in frustration as you ask yourself a most
excellent question: "Why didn't I get into great shape years ago?!"

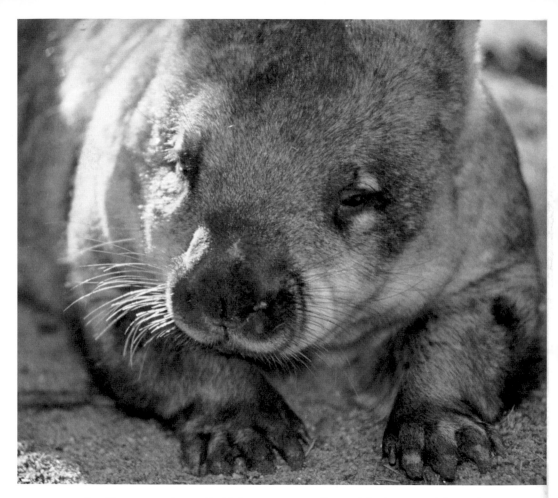

So there you have it. Unless you can live with the anguish and responsibility of being sleek, slim, and svelte, you may well be better off staying an idle, plump, dissatisfied dumpling living in perpetual denial.

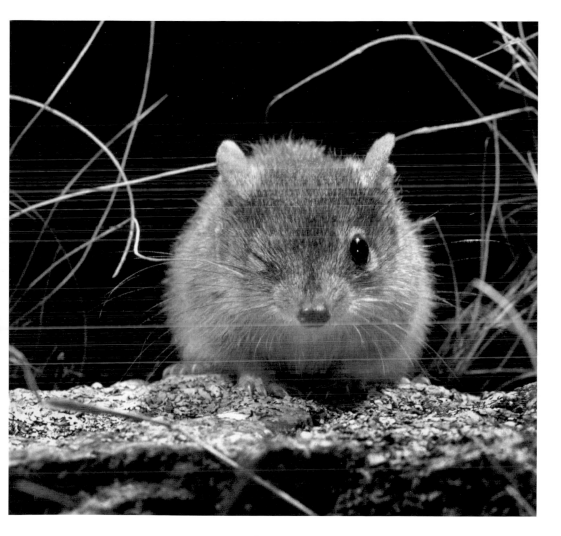

Or not.

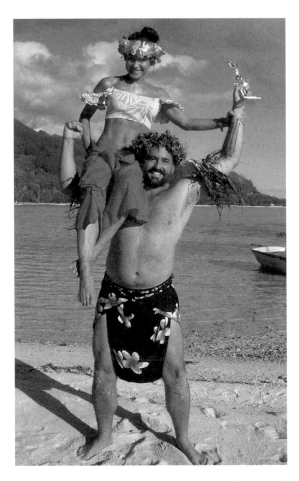

Bradley Trevor Greive, for a time "the world's strongest author of amusing little gift books," celebrates his 2005 Regional Rock-Lifting Championship in Ha'apiti, French Polynesia, with a local lovely. Flush with victory and French pastries, BTG went on to bulk up his bookish beefcake until his traditional Polynesian pareu (sarong) was the only thing he could wear without rupturing a zipper—
hence, this book . . .